Life in-out

No ~~Emotions,~~ It's all about SMART BALANCING

UTTAM KUMAR

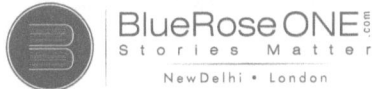

BLUEROSE PUBLISHERS
India | U.K.

Copyright © Uttam Kumar 2025

All rights reserved by author. No part of this publication may be reproduced, stored in a retrieval system or transmitted in any form or by any means, electronic, mechanical, photocopying, recording or otherwise, without the prior permission of the author. Although every precaution has been taken to verify the accuracy of the information contained herein, the publisher assumes no responsibility for any errors or omissions. No liability is assumed for damages that may result from the use of information contained within.

BlueRose Publishers takes no responsibility for any damages, losses, or liabilities that may arise from the use or misuse of the information, products, or services provided in this publication.

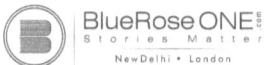

For permissions requests or inquiries regarding this publication, please contact:

BLUEROSE PUBLISHERS
www.BlueRoseONE.com
info@bluerosepublishers.com
+91 8882 898 898
+4407342408967

ISBN: 978-93-6783-141-0

Cover Design: Shubham Verma
Typesetting: Sagar

First Edition: May 2025

Introduction

Today, we are all facing a world which is quite different from the past. The disintegration of the joint family and the development of urbanization gave rise to such a brand of individualism, where even a single person has developed the idea that if he wants, he can achieve everything on the basis of his hard work. He can withstand the pressure of competition to stay ahead at the professional level. He can maintain interpersonal relationships by keeping himself at the center. He can adjust one's image as per the needs of social media. If you need advice, social media, the internet, or a life coach can fix it in a moment. There is just one price to be paid for this – sacrificing your mental health and physical fitness.

For the last twenty years, I have deeply studied the lifestyle of people living around me, especially their thinking pattern and their communication models. It is these two that determine the quality of our entire life. The whole universe, like any other system, functions on the input-output model: "what comes in, will go out". The guiding principle here is "equilibrium" or the universal balance of energy. Its quantity will always be the same, but it can be changed in many forms, depending upon the thought process and communication maturity by which the three players of life – self, other selves, and the universe – balance themselves.

Energy is the only natural raw material provided to us by the universe, whose final product or output is thought. As long as this thought is one's internal matter or till it does not come out, it will not disturb or unbalance others. But it will keep its creator or producer unbalanced, which may result in mental (anger, anxiety, pain, or stress, restlessness), physical (various lifestyle diseases), or cultural (social unrest, riots) imbalance. It has to come out rationally to make a useful balance. So, if possible, live without generating any thoughts, which is impossible as long as you are human.

Once the idea is generated, it now becomes an input for you, which has to be transformed into an output in the form of "action" or "communication". Your actions or task implementation style and communication skills then become inputs for others. These inputs have the potential to make you balanced or unbalanced through three different responses – support, challenge, or indifference. This is why in today's life our actions and communication patterns are regularly questioned - "Why did you do that?" "Why didn't you do that?", "Is that the way to talk to me?" or otherwise - "Good job or thanks or it doesn't matter to me." And it is now the responsibility of others to establish or ensure balance.

In practice, this hardly happens and hence there are so many ills in our social and personal lives. In fact, whatever you think or do is to balance yourself, which does not mean that others also get balanced at the same time. This is true for everyone and every society which makes us believe that if there is life, there will be problems. We all have to struggle hard or compete with others to achieve success. Think positive, stay away from negative people, and stay committed to your goal, and you will attract the same, or the universe will give you what you want. All these may be slogans of a mid-life crisis, reached at this stage without studying the starting and end point of life, which is peace and cooperation. Today's cut-throat competition and intolerance have never been a part of life, and perhaps due to the intrusions of these alien ideas in our mind, we experience the resultant stress and anxiety, adversely affecting the quality of life and also the maximum happiness of the maximum people.

This book is therefore based on ideas of bringing balance and peace into everyone's life through its three parts – Thought, Balance, and Communication – which evolve around a single key statement – "Balanced thought expressed through balanced communication". Thought means the unity of ideas without contradictions, the principle of balance, supported by logic and science, and communication in the form of linguistic monism. These three processes are like yogic pranayama. How much we inhale (take), how long we hold it and how much we exhale (give out).

To live a peaceful and balanced life we are generally advised to refine our thought process, which determines our actions and according to which we bring about results for ourselves in this world. But should this be the starting point of reform? This thought process has always been as undefined and abstract as Shankaracharya's "Brahman". It is relatively difficult for an average person to start from here. It is like finding gold in sand dunes. So, don't exert yourself too much. You can easily find them in your daily interactions rather than in thought. Only condition is to watch out for your communication pattern with your utmost awareness.

In fact, communication and thought are inseparable. All thoughts are inherently tied to communication. Communication is not just a tool for expressing pre-existing ideas, but it also shapes and determines the way we think through constant interaction. This approach implies that our understanding of the world and our ideas about it are constrained or heavily influenced by the structure and limitations of our communication patterns. This book is therefore intended to engage all those involved in any form of communication and to provide readily available tools through which we can continually refine our thinking in order to achieve the ultimate balance.

The importance of this book lies in its ability to inspire, educate, and equip elders, teens and younger generations with the tools they need to find balance in the world to live a more balanced and fulfilling life in any situation.

Life is not a struggle but cooperation. There is no misery or problems in life, but happiness and peace. The only prerequisite is to comprehend nature properly. This very comprehension is wisdom. It is the attainment of supreme knowledge and enlightenment. Therefore, we need to turn the direction of our thought this way. We have to see things as non-dual or 'One'. We have to understand the difference between 'what is being shown' and 'what should be shown'. What that is 'one' has been shown as two or many from time immemorial. Then an attempt is made to comprehend it. If we construe 'one' as 'two', we will definitely get perplexed. Now we must struggle to work on this confusion so that it can be re-understood as one. Such as, we tend to create confusion by first dividing the pure idea into many parts, just as we divide a pure person into negatives and positives. When this misleading information creates a problem, we suggest a way to turn towards positive thoughts or positive persons. We intend to get people entangled in the duality of success and failure. Many such ideas have been implanted in our existence that keep our lives busy in struggling to achieve a purpose that nowhere exists. This is the reason why almost all, after achieving one's cherished ambition, get dissatisfied at some point of time and restart to achieve yet another goal that they themselves don't know. This continues till our life is over or we attain this wisdom. To be precise, life has become like making 'one' into 'two' and then struggling to make 'two' into 'one'. However, most lives start from 'two' and end with two, struggling throughout and claiming that 'Life is nothing but struggle' or that 'life and problems coexist'. So, this book makes you enlightened enough from the very beginning by letting you know 'one' is 'one' and only then you can enjoy the human construct 'twos'.

In many literatures, the responsibility of these confusions is put on the mind by saying that the mind is fickle, the mind is unstable, the mind is weak, and the mind is strong. The mind is neither weak, nor fickle, nor unstable, nor strong. It is nothing but a motion, only as it has to be like that due to its very nature of being dynamic. Due to this very nature, it generates energy on its own with which it sustains its existence as well as the existence of its temporary shelters, i. e. our body, and thereby the entire Universe. It is our duty to recombine the energy into the right combination. Do not blame your mind for not doing so and thus absolve yourself of all your responsibilities. Trying to become a doctor is like usurping the designated role of the universal supreme. You are only a compounder, and the mind is only a supplier of as much energy as you require. So don't be greedy or miserly. The right amount of energy in the right proportion is medicine. So, consume it in the right quantity, neither less nor more. This way you make your time come, and that will make you what you want to be.

The first part of this book, "Thought," is an attempt to promote such a different or alternate way of thinking so that we can understand that life is not a struggle but cooperation. Life is not a misery or problems, but happiness and peace. There is nothing in nature, neither a life nor a substance is too much or too less. We call this situation a balance that is capable of maintaining the existence of any existence. A person or a substance is not going to move even an inch from its original position if any kind of imbalance does not arise.

This imbalance can be physical, mental, or cultural. The dynamics of physical balance and imbalance find a place in Newton's third law of motion-"For every action, there is an equal and opposite reaction". This implies that a body or matter naturally balances itself, and it happens too. If a person abuses us, it also means that he makes us mentally unbalanced. We regain our mental balance by abusing him back or by choosing some other options. We certainly do. All the erstwhile imperialist powers of the world have been using the dynamics of mental imbalance-balance to fulfill their political interests. The British ruled India for a long time using this very dynamics unsparingly. For centuries, human society has been establishing its cultural balance by bringing changes in itself according to the demands of the time from time to time to maintain its existence.

In this sense, the authority of balance is paramount and supreme. It is sovereign in the real sense. In the entire process of evolution of mankind, different periods witnessed the emergence of thought or idea among humans of becoming sovereign by amassing unsurmountable power and authority. This disturbed the concept of collective balance in such a way that none of our generations had a look back from here again. First, this collective balance was disturbed by the incursion of personal whims. This led to the emergence of a myriad of problems. This necessitated fighting these problems and life became another name for struggle, unrest, misery, and problems. People started being taught and trained to fight it. Weapons like anger, hatred, hostility, fear, happiness, humor, etc. were presented in the guise of emotions to achieve the desired state. This desired state is actually a state of peace or balance. But has anyone been able to achieve this state? We are all simply living our lives in the name of struggle. That is, the start and end point of life have been accepted as nothing but struggle instead of peace. It seems that the chapter on peace and cooperation has been marginalized from the core syllabus of life and prioritized over struggle and cut-throat competition. Children are struggling with studies, youths are struggling for jobs, the quadragenarians are struggling for their livelihood, and the elderly are struggling for physical health. All this made me write the second part of this book "Balance" with the intention to facilitate us to choose those ideological choices that are always available to us so as to achieve a state of balance or a rudimentary state of peace.

In whatever way we know the life or nature, its sole source is thought. Whether it is created by ourselves, perceived through our sense organs or it is created by supporting or disagreeing with the ideas advanced by others or co-humans. Whether we believe in any of those thoughts or not, or whether we act thereon or not, depends on the extent to which we are imbalanced by those thoughts. This does not mean that we are, as our thoughts are. It is only as much as we are able to express our thoughts through our actions and our daily conversations. This conversation can be between self and self through the process of introspection or between self and others through interaction. Hence, it is easy for us to conclude that the main source of our physical, mental and cultural makeup or problems is the daily conversations that we have.

Hence, the third and last part of this book is titled 'Communication'. This is where the treasure of life is hidden. It's here, where thoughts are created, from where thoughts enter inside us, and from where our thoughts go out so that the desired balance can be achieved or endorsing the cyclical system "Whatever comes has to go out". This is the platform where our life seeks the possibility of remaining balanced through action-reaction dynamics. For example, the reason for our physical and mental problems can be that we make someone our enemy in our mind and keep planning to take revenge on him throughout our lives. In the end, it turns out that there was nothing like that. We may have differences with someone or the other at our workplace. This increases our stress level to any extent. This will definitely have an adverse impact on our physical and mental health. So it is our unwavering belief that if we pay attention to our daily conversations and follow the process mentioned in this book, we will find that by keeping ourselves as well as others balanced in our conversations, we can make the overall energy flow towards us. This will help us to achieve cent percent success in whatever we yearn for in life.

Through this book, I am suggesting that you adopt a new system of medicine or treatment. This medicine system is communication therapy. There is no need to do any additional practice for this. All you have to do is, whenever you talk to someone, you remind yourself that you are in the process of healing. Every word that comes from the other side, every sentence spoken by you, and the conclusion that you draw from the conversation is a medicine or Doctor's prescription for you. This medicine may work for you, but it may also have contraindications for you, and it may also cause adverse drug reactions. The expiry date of the medicine also has to be kept in mind. If you are so alert in your daily conversations, believe me, you can free yourself from all the diseases that are caused by anxiety and stress. You will agree that most of the diseases we get are due to the anxiety and stress that we take in through various pathways of life.

Students can study with full concentration while undergoing this treatment process. They can be successful in competitive exams. Parents can save their children from the ill-effects of modern gadgets, distractions, and bad company by being in this healing process. We can touch new heights of success at our workplace by giving better dimensions to inter-personal relations with our officers, our colleagues and our subordinates. Ultimately, by striking harmony and balance with ourselves, our family, and society, we can experience the much-required peace that is envisioned in that chapter of life which is never taught but lived.

New Delhi/Kolkata

Uttam Kumar

April 2025

Dedication

Dedicated to my late beloved parents

Although you are no longer here, your love, wisdom, and unwavering encouragement continue to guide my path. Your enduring belief in my dreams energizes my journey every day. This book is a tribute to the invaluable lessons you have taught me by your example—resilience, compassion, and the pursuit of greatness. Your legacy lives on in every word written and every life touched.

Forever in my heart,

Uttam Kumar

Acknowledgement

To my beloved wife and the light of my life, my precious 9-year-old daughter,

As I embark on this journey of discovery into the intricate fabric of inspiration, I am destined to dedicate these words to two of the most inspiring personalities in my world. My dear wife, your unwavering support and boundless love have been my anchor through the storms and the wind beneath the wings of my aspirations. In your gaze, I find the inspiration to transcend limits and strive for greatness, knowing that your love is my strongest foundation.

My dear daughter, you have already become the embodiment of joy and curiosity. Your infectious laughter and innocent wonder fuel my determination to create a world full of endless possibilities for you. As I write thoughts on motivation, I am reminded that every forward-looking inspiration is rooted in the desire to create a brighter future for you, where dreams are not only cherished but pursued with unwavering passion.

This book is a testament to how deeply you both have impacted my life. May its pages continue to resonate with the same love, encouragement, and inspiration that you have generously showered upon me. Here's to my source of inspiration, my wife and daughter, who make every step of this journey worthwhile.

Further, all through the journey of my writing, my Father-in-law and Mother-in law remained with me like a beacon. It was all like the role, ricocheted from my parents to them by divine-like inheritance.

My sincere thanks to my cousin, Gunjan Sahaa, who was thoroughly critical of my thought and helped me to develop the entire plot of my book. He single-handedly designed the title page. I also acknowledge the service of Dineshwar Kumar Sah, Artist, Botanical Survey of India, who has inserted beautiful sketches, thereby adding value and life to the book.

Uttam Kumar

For Readers

Dear Reader,

Welcome to a journey of self-discovery and transformation—a journey that explores the incredible power that lies in your thoughts and communication. This book is a guidebook destined to help you navigate the complex landscapes of your mind, promote thought, balance, and refine your communication skills. In our daily lives, our thoughts often shape our reality, influencing our actions and relationships. It is important to understand the deep impact of our thoughts and how they manifest in our communication. This book aims to unravel the complexities of this relationship, offering insights and practical strategies for harnessing the potential of balanced thinking and balanced communication.

The purpose here is not to confuse you with the duality of negativity or positivity of thoughts, but rather to bring harmony to your mind, recognizing the thoughts that serve you and those that hinder your growth. Through introspection and guidance, you will discover ways to develop a healthier mental landscape, empowering yourself to face the demands of life with resilience and optimism.

Communication is the bridge that connects us to the world. How we express our thoughts shapes our interactions and relationships. This book sheds light on the art of balanced communication, highlighting the nuances of active listening, empathy, non-verbal cues, and assertiveness. By honing these skills, you will discover your ability to express yourself authentically and connect more deeply with others. It may be noted that the words communication and conversation have been used in different parts of this book in the same sense.

As you embark on this journey, remember that change is a gradual process. Each chapter presents an opportunity for growth and reflection. The exercises and principles shared here are tools designed to accompany you on your path toward personal and interpersonal growth. It is advisable not to read this book in one sitting. After reading each paragraph, pause. Reflect. Relate it to your own life. Then only you can move on.

I encourage you to approach this book with an open mind and a willingness to embrace change. Embrace the power of balanced thoughts and balanced communication and see how it transforms not only your interactions with others but also your relationship with yourself. This is where you gain the confidence to achieve whatever you are striving for.

Hope this book will serve as a guide in your journey towards the balance of thought and balanced communication.

Best wishes for this transformative campaign.

Contents

Part I: THOUGHT 1
- If a Wasp Bites You, Celebrate 5
- Thought is Thought: Neither
  Negative nor Positive 11
- Being in Grief is A Loss of Many Joys 19
- Everyone is Successful 25
- Moving is Becoming 33
- Break a Glass Everyday 39
- Problem: New Version of Old Solution 45
- If Anger is Bound to Come,
  Invest & Encash 51
- The More Nervous You Are,
  The More Scientific You Are 65
- First Question: Leads you to lead 71

PART-II: BALANCE 79
- Law of Return- Parting, Knowing
  and Returning 80
- Knowing- Life is just a continuum of
  Balance and Imbalance 83

- To Return is to Join: Where and How? 90
- Authority of Balance 97
- The Basic Nature of Life: Peace. Dropdown Theory 101
- Principle of Balance: Some Stories from My Life 118

PART-III: COMMUNICATION 129
1. Type B Stage: 137
2. Type V Stage: 159
3. Type H Stage: 166

Author's Note: Key Takeaways

Part I

Thought

Thought is the first product of man which is created from the transformation of energy received from the universe. Its movement or entry and exit can be from both ends. From thought to action or from action to thought. It is a difficult task for an average human being to grasp thoughts directly. It would be good if people take care of the words, they use in their daily communication because these words give expression to the thoughts they have already formed and also provide inputs or raw material for the formation of future thoughts. So your dialogue and the words used in it will keep you fully aware of the process of idea formation and again, its usage according to time and space. For example, one person brings vegetables from the market and keeps them in the refrigerator. The other person cooks the vegetables after a few days. The vegetables may lose their freshness by then. The person who eats them may not like the taste and there is a high probability that he will criticize them, if not in front, behind the back, or in mind. The second situation is when a person who brings fresh vegetables from the market, himself cooks and eats them immediately, then there is a high probability that he will enjoy their taste properly. It means, the one who is involved in the process or understands the process will also make better use of the product.

The purpose of putting thoughts in the first part of this book is that since our early life, we have been told that a person should have high thoughts because whatever our thoughts are, so will our actions be. It has been said that whatever you think, so will you be. You can either agree or disagree with this. In my opinion, it is not true that you are what you think. I believe that you become what you do. You do something only when you know that it is right or that it can be done. It is not that you do only, what you think because when you do it is not the result of your thought alone. The thoughts of that time clash with your previous thoughts and time and circumstances limit you. And in this way, you keep changing. You express yourself in different forms in different circumstances. You are a specific person to someone when someone catches you in a certain situation. So, first of all, we have taken ten popular ideas which have influenced the direction of our life. This idea is very important for us because of the way it has been used, it can be used in other ways also. If this happens then it will be very easy for us to see life in its true sense because with such thinking or idea, we will be able to connect things with ourselves, other selves like us, and the universe in a balanced manner.

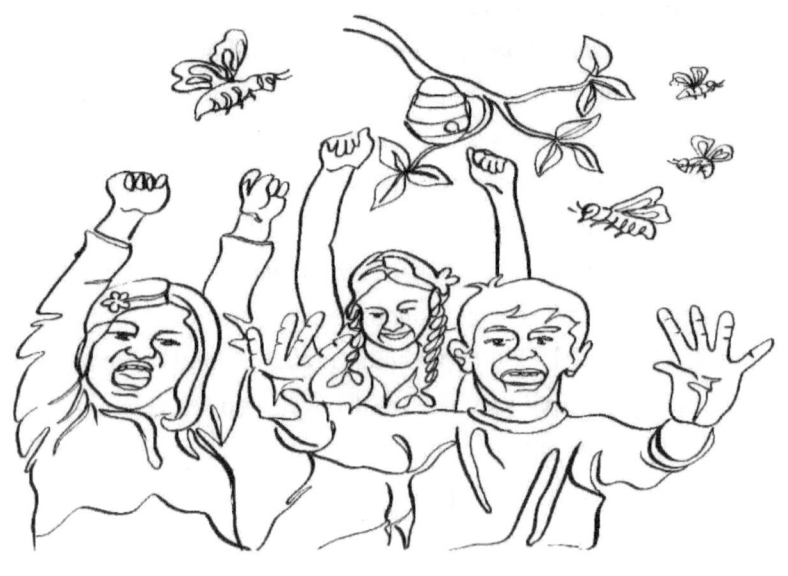

If a Wasp Bites You, Celebrate

As a principal of a residential academic institution in Punjab, I had to face a unique issue. In the month of April-May, the wasps started moving around to make their nests, and during this time many students were seen complaining every day that the wasps had stung them badly and their entire face got swollen. I was very much perturbed and down because as their head I could not solve their issue. But the surprising thing for me was why that wasp was not stinging me. I also wanted to have that experience. I told the same to our children. Perhaps they liked my empathy. I held a group meeting and appealed to all that from now whenever a wasp bites, we have to thank it and celebrate because through this, it has taught us a wonderful lesson and inspired us.

Let us change the direction. Now, try to see from the point of view of the wasp. It targeted us and we became its prey. In this way, wasps succeeded in achieving their objective and it was we who could not manage to escape. In place, without wasting time, we directly blamed the wasps for this. The result was that we always failed to defend ourselves. As long as we keep saying that we are bitten by a dog, stung by a snake, or gored by a bull, these things will keep happening to us because we will expect them to change. Will they change? If not, again be ready to get the things repeated. Get a fact-checked, it is a part of their nature or a method of self-defence, rightly used by them. Then why should we even think about it? It is so simple – it was we who had to try to defend ourselves.

Whenever we think outside of ourselves, as we do, particularly if something bad happens to us, in the language of physics, we move away from the center of mass. In the same way, we move away from the solution too to that extent. Only when we start taking responsibility for ourselves, will we be able to think about improvement, and appropriate improvement will also take place. The responsibility of not taking responsibility has been our age-old rite. For example, from our very childhood we have been taught in English grammar that, during the use of the article 'the', there are some eternal or universal truths like "The Sun rises in the east and sets in the west". Whereas the truth is that we move with the rotation of the Earth. The sun remains relatively still. When we are in front of the sun, it is bright and when we move away from the sun, it is dark. Now whose responsibility is it? Of Sun or of ours? It is like this, if we fall into darkness, it is the responsibility of the Sun that it has set, and if we are on the brighter side, then also it is the responsibility of the Sun that it has risen. Now the sun has to answer why it rose and why it set.

We can call these statements linguistic tricks. What difference does it make if we say that we were stung by a wasp or that we could not escape? The difference decides the approach that we are supposed to take. Further, if both statements can be used interchangeably, then why should not other approaches be adopted? This will not happen because it is completely scientific that man will be selfish. Whenever he thinks, he will keep himself in the center and the responsibility will be to someone else. To be freed from responsibility in this way is to become inert, which is a natural property of the matter or body. This is because we consider the mind as the body and react accordingly. If the philosophy or mind-set is body or matter oriented then all the scientific laws that apply to matter will apply to us and we will say that "a wasp stung us" and if the philosophy or mind-set is mind-based, we will proceed to acquire all the desired human qualities and will say "we could not escape".

Whenever something untoward happens to you, definitely think about your role in it. You will find that at some places you yourself are responsible and will try to bring appropriate improvements in it. I would like to tell you that I stayed there for almost two years thereafter, but the wasp was never able to prey on me. There could be two probable reasons for this. One was that I was always waiting for it to come. When you are waiting for someone, you are preparing yourself for the situation that may arise from their arrival. This way you are able to negotiate the impending situation successfully. On the contrary, when we complain, it means that we are neither prepared for it nor do we want to contribute to its improvement. For example, we often complain that the exam did not go well because the question paper was difficult. Complaining is a function of these two causes.

Complaining or shifting the responsibility elsewhere is such a habit that the one who has fallen prey to it can never recover. Unfortunately, a person does not even realize how slowly he sacrifices his personality. There comes a time when he starts complaining about himself and finds himself at a dead end. This is because he has always tried in this direction only and trying is also a kind of habit.

———————————

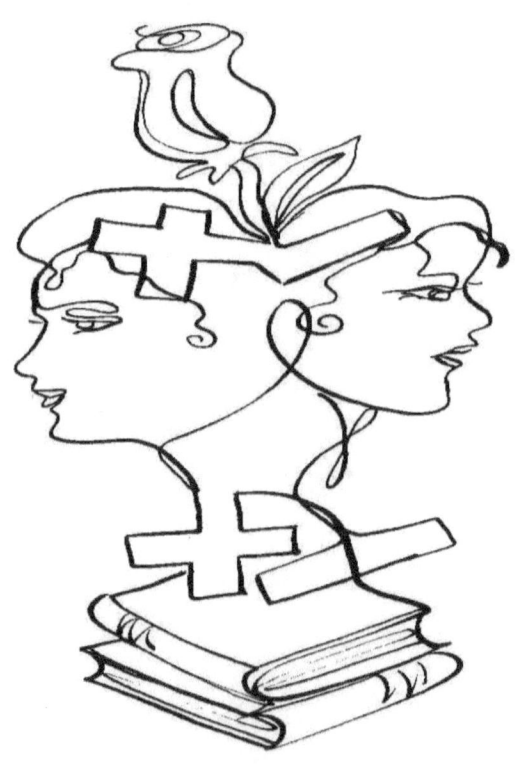

Thought is Thought: Neither Negative nor Positive

This idea may seem to be queer to you, but it is true. You will soon realize that you have never looked at the idea or perspective from this perspective before. It is important how we look at something. When our perspective changes, the process of formation of our nature starts, as does our reaction. I do not want to get into the controversy of negative or positive thinking or thought here. Thoughts cannot be negative or positive. Thoughts are thoughts, which are relative to time and space and people make them so according to their convenience. The same is the case with negative or positive attitudes or negative or positive people. If we start seeing ourselves as a factor of any incident (or accident), the ideology of negative or positive thought or attitude or person comes to its doom.

Our valuable time is wasted in arguing whether his thoughts are negative or positive. Or whether a particular person is negative or positive, or whether his attitude is negative or positive. In fact, whenever we say this, we move away from ourselves, and the more we move away from ourselves, the more we move away from the solution too. Is there any permanent measure on the basis of which we can classify any thought or person, or attitude as negative or positive? Or you can prepare a list of 100 thoughts or persons, or attitudes that are definitely negative or positive. For example, "destruction" is a negative word, so shouldn't suffering be destroyed? Words or thoughts are just nouns "denoting" words that can be used differently in different situations.

We hesitate to be a part of any incident because there is a sense of responsibility there-in. We can easily say that I do not want to meet a particular person because he is negative. If he is positive, it may challenge our status quo. I am fine the way I am. I don't want to start a new venture by calling anyone positive. Getting into this kind of duel would be like taking on the burden of extra work. First, the person is already disturbed, and he is told not to think negatively, but rather to think positively. Now, prepare a list of negative words or persons or visualize. Sort out the word or person that is incompatible with it. Then try to stay away from it or whatever. So you are being burdened with additional tasks. You don't have to get into these things. Instead try to seize the idea or the person in its primordial form where it originates.

Being shown half a bucket of water, I may be asked how I see this bucket. If I answer that the bucket is half full, I will be judged as a positive thinker or positive person. Saying the bucket is half empty, I am put in the category of a negative thinker or negative person. Science has its own version, the bucket cannot be empty as it is filled with air. If I say the whole bucket is empty, then I am a person with an extremely negative attitude. If I say the whole bucket is empty and it will be filled with all my hard work, then how should it be seen? Until we appreciate the emptiness, there will be no attempt to fill it. Looking at emptiness promotes and strengthens the process of envisioning and carving out a space for creativity and innovation. So the question is not whether there is a deficiency or void here, the question is that yes, there is a deficit here and what can I do to fill it. So, it should be assumed that first, we have to be negative and then positive. This negative/positive exercise is initiated by those who enjoy being comfortable in debate. For the doer, it is only a situation, and he decides what his role is, in improvising the condition.

If a person is considered negative, or if he is like that. Or let's say that person is negative. If at any point in time, that person is saying something beneficial to society. What will be the reaction of the people? How will the public take it? Generally, it will be said that the person should first look at himself and then preach. This means that because that person is negative, he cannot say anything good to the public. It may be decoded in this way too. Since we cannot support good things, it would be better if we talk about their character. The question is simple—if a dishonest person is saying good things and it is good for everyone, then what is the harm in believing him? Why do we waste time in evaluating his character? Then there are many such stories, and legends that have nothing to do with reality but inspire us. So shouldn't these be adopted? Some people are in the habit of naming wonderful ideas as good philosophy but impractical, so that they should not be forced to apply this in their lives. In fact, it is the nature of matter to confine itself to the least space so that it does not have to expend much energy. For this, we will have to do less work, just like the raindrop becomes round or the law of octet in chemistry, which forces our body to be inert.

This is why giving advice, seeking advice or accepting advice is like a strategy whose evaluation depends on the effect it has on us.

Let's simplify the things with an example. We have to buy tomatoes from the vegetable market. Will we see whether the tomato seller looks handsome and smart? Or is he a liar? Or will we see who has good tomatoes? Even after being satisfied with this, we will sort out the tomatoes to see which ones are good. Here it is important to see that we have selected only the good tomatoes. But when we get an opportunity to meet a person, we tend to sort out only his/her shortcomings. We hardly try to develop our personality by adopting his/her qualities.

Now let's talk about the dynamics of positivity and negativity with the help of the same vegetable market. Here we assume that positive or negative thinking is not in the picture. While sorting tomatoes, you might not have selected tomatoes that were either unripe or overripe. You had to buy some unripe tomatoes so that they could be used for the next few days. That's why you bought some unripe tomatoes. At the same time, a person standing next to you is selecting overripe tomatoes because he has to make tomato chutney for a wedding. Here, the person selling tomatoes, the price of tomatoes, the time, and the market are constant, but the selection process has changed. Hence, a personality should not be defined by adjectives like positive or negative based on the mere selection process.

I never looked at my life in a positive or negative sense at any level. I found myself in a situation, tried to understand it, and responded accordingly, and whatever the result was, made it the basis for the next course of action.

Despite all these, if you are bound to believe that there are negative or positive words or people, then they should accept that such a situation arises when you or like-minded are highly subjective and see the time and situation through the lens of their own making. Barring a few exceptions, all the people you see in this world are mixed packs of energy. If we talk about Indian philosophy, there is a combination of Satva, Tamas, and Rajas. If we talk about science, we have black, we have yellow, we have blue, and what not, if we go by thousands of color shades. But when you mix all of them, you find it white. So we find a person in combinations. It is the responsibility of society to see the white color behind these and try to enhance those colors that are in the interest of society. Our society has never been free from this responsibility. This world belongs to all of us. We should try to stay away from these superfluous engagements and accept the principle of diversity of nature and fulfil this responsibility from the smallest unit of society, to all of us via family. This kind of thinking will free you from unnecessary distractions and give you much-needed time to concentrate on your desired goal.

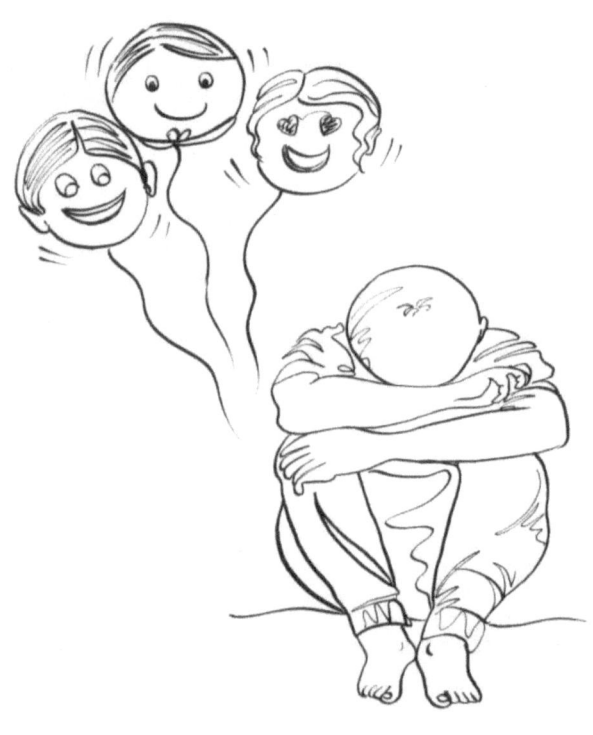

Being in Grief is a Loss of Many Joys

You are in grief. It means that something bad or very bad has happened to you. It has happened to you only. No one is with you. Certainly not your close ones. Some appear to be on your side or may not be, some out of pity, and some are with genuine intent. But your grief cannot be their grief because they, too, have their own. It is your personal property which can be discussed but cannot never be transferred. To be in grief means to contemplate grief, trying to identify its reasons and to continue to dump into it as if it is a mystery and one has to delve deep into it to make out its character. And the more you dive into it, the more likely you are to get into it and in the end, you will fetch the same for yourself.

Grief is a consciously chosen response to a situation in which you are uncomfortable, and you use your power and energy elsewhere. How bad has happened to you will depend on how much you thought about an issue and how much you got it. Being good or bad may be a part of the dictionary of business, not of life. Life is life, and to drive it, you need a good driver who crosses all the mountains, plains, rivers, forests, and dangers on the way and reaches his destination. The farther the journey, the more you get these.

If you want to travel a long distance by train, then obviously you prefer to travel by express train because you have to reach early. It will not stop at small stations. But this does not mean that these small stations will disappear. They will remain at their places, but you will not stop there. Passenger trains will stop at every small and big station, they will reach their destination late but they will definitely reach. Life is like this. Those that may not be your destination, may not even be a part of your thoughts, still you will face them. It just depends on how long you take a halt and where you stop. Air travel will take you from one place to another in a few minutes. But you cannot enjoy the beauty en route. The higher you fly, the more you get away from its truth. If you have to travel by sea, you will have to endure the storms and the waves. Can you imagine a steady ship? If yes, then it will be found only on the riverside and seashore. Dry, stumpy, and useless, and it may be infested with termites that have the potential to erase all its evidence. The existence of a ship means that it can move forward by maintaining its balance while negotiating the waves of the sea. This is life and has to be travelled by all modes of transport.

Besides, we are human beings, with a vacillating mind and a relaxed body, so we are either in a hurry or are relatively late, but nature is always on time. So, if nothing is going your way despite your best efforts, please understand that either you are late or the time is yet to come. Stay calm and keep doing simple tasks. When circumstances are not favorable to you, you only encounter the reasons for their absence and it leads to problems in the future. Some people feel that nothing is going to happen in their life now, as if there will never be a morning after the night. Spending the night in distress is indeed a big challenge. But you will see that you fall into a deep sleep in the first part of the morning, and when you open your eyes, it is already daytime. Being in grief is the loss of many joys. You lost your delicious breakfast. It means that when you are sad, you get entangled in all the reasons that make you sad, while at the same time, many good things are happening around you or could have happened. During that period, you did not watch any good movies. You did not go for a walk with friends or family. You did not study anything. You did not remember any good event that happened in your life in the past or any good omen that was to come, and when good times came, you realized that you were thinking in vain. The dilemma during the interregnum between the exam is over and the announcement of results in the life of the student can be easily understood. But after getting entangled in unexpected thoughts and losing good moments, even if the exam result is good, another problem arises. I was thinking uselessly. And during this time, I lost this.

Whatever is there good or bad, let it be happened. It has to happen and it will happen. This universe also has some plans which may not suit you but serve a bigger purpose and may be in your own interest as a part of the common good. You just concentrate on the final purpose. The process of making the product and the final product are two different things. A serious problem will arise if we put the two in the place of each other. The food being cooked, the house being built, the statue being sculpted, and the pictures being drawn are not their final products. Therefore, our reaction should also be similar. In the same way, accepting a few selected incidents of life as the ultimate truth of life would be like accepting the process as the final product. And here, since the question itself is based on this illusion, the answer will surely confuse.

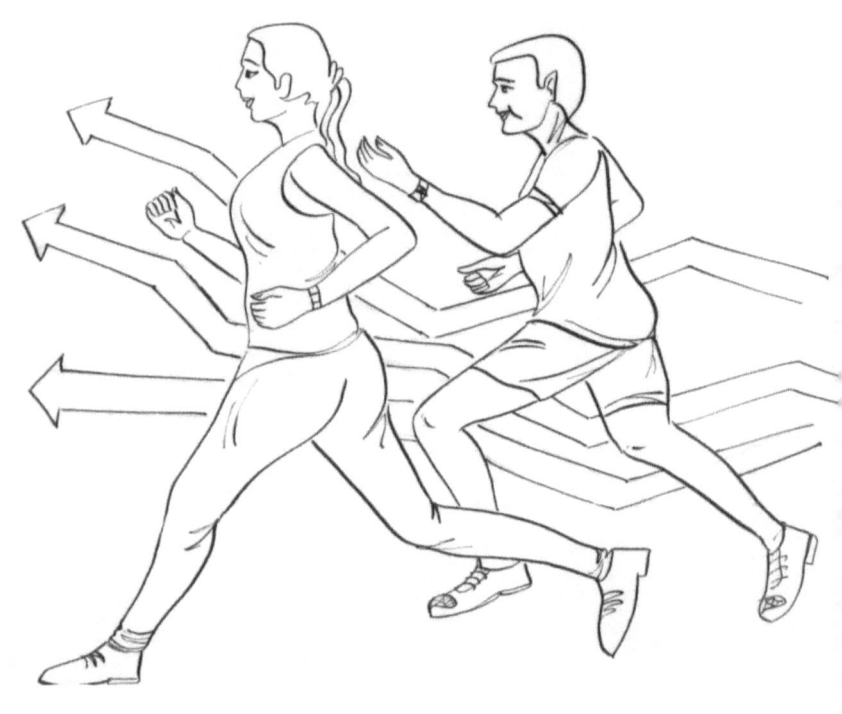

Everyone is Successful

I have not seen any unsuccessful or failed person in my life to date. In my opinion, a person never fails. He just awards terms to that stage of work or effort of his own volition, where he feels so uncomfortable and incapable of making further attempts. He feels that he has suffered a loss there. The other way round, if you look at the things in which you have benefited even a little? Then you will find that in that situation also you must have been benefited in some way or the other. If not, at least you have done some work whose good results may be hidden in the womb of the future.

In fact, the idea that failure is a pillar of success is self-contradictory. If failure is a step towards success, then reaching that step is also a success. Therefore, every step of ours takes us to some destination. Hence, there is no need to be disappointed, but we have to take another take off from there with new vigor and energy.

If we want to reach the sun and get tired after reaching the moon, it does not mean that we have failed. We are in a better position than before and have reached a new level. Now either one moves further or someone else will take a start from here. This is the mandatory pathway of all kinds of development.

Everywhere a person keeps saying that he is not satisfied, there is a want, deficiency, or problem in his life. This is because he does not think about what he has; he thinks about what he does not have. In this way, you develop a habit of thinking about what you do not have, which slowly takes the form of a permanent tendency. Another side of such people is that they do not see the deprivations in the lives of others. It's like I have nothing, but others have. So, it can be said that everyone has everything. So think what others think of you. In this way, I have a lot, but others lack a lot. Then see what kind of nature develops within you, and you will find yourself richer and stronger than others, and this will generate a new energy, and you will move ahead.

Once Narad ji was taking a round of the Earth. Many people complained that they did not have anything. They don't get what they desire. This made Narad ji very sad. After reaching Vishnu Lok, he asked Lord Vishnu, Lord, people on the Earth are very unhappy. They do not get what they want. Everyone is hopeless. Vishnu ji said that it is not so, I have equipped humans with all those qualities so that they can get whatever they want. Narad Ji prayed, "Lord, still you should do something for them." Whenever they get unhappy, they say that it is God's will, which makes you defamed which is unbearable for me. Under pressure, Lord Vishnu gave a big bag to Naradji and directed him to make copies of it and distribute it among all the people. Tell them that whatever one wants, one should just look into this bag and one will certainly get it. Narada ji was very happy. He immediately went down and distributed the bag to each and every inhabitant of the earth and said that whatever you want, look inside this bag and ask for it, you will get it.

After a year, Narad ji revisited the Earth hoping to see everyone happy. But what he saw was that they had become poorer than before. A committee was formed to find out what wrong had happened to them. It was found that instead of looking into one's own bag, everyone kept trying to peep into the bag of others to see what the other person got. One could never see one's own bag. They could never make themselves understand what exactly they wanted. So should it be understood that at least they understood what everyone else wanted? Such things are found in our society. I wish you could look at yourself once, and try to understand yourself. Then you will feel that there is everything in this world that you can get. The conclusion is that we have to make a habit of first thinking about what we have and then using it as a resource to touch new heights. Nothing has been created from nothing and neither will it be created. So, if you keep thinking about 'nothing', you will always get nothing. Then how do you say that you did not get what you thought? Whatever we think, whatever we want, we definitely get it if we execute our plan accordingly. Thinking is the first step only, not the final step. It will only lead your mind to work on options based on the inputs available, aiming at ultimate accomplishment. You keep thinking that you will get fewer marks in the exam, and you get less marks. So, celebrate it because you got what you thought, then why to lament?

No person can fail. Success demands solid practice. Besides, it is relative. If a student does not study for years and fails in the exam, it does not mean that he has failed. In fact, he was prepared not to succeed in the exam by not studying for years and failed in the exam, hence he succeeded. In fact, if you prepare for failure, you will achieve success in it. Apart from this, due to the fear of failure, a student prays to God that he should not fail or prays again and again, "O, God let me pass this test." The fear of failure works in the background. In this way, the energy of failure will dominate his entire psyche. So do not get into this ideological conflict and keep working. Just like the way a whole house can be built by placing bricks one after another. Thinking about it only will encourage the tendency to think only, and action on it becomes difficult. Then there is also the fear of time slipping from the hand. It is better once the objective is clear, think about its smaller units and act on them. Gradually, you will see that you have reached your destination. To achieve a big objective, it is necessary to divide it into smaller units and celebrate each part after completing it. If you have to go a hundred miles, then you start and see that after completing each step, you take the next step with double enthusiasm. It has become our habit that instead of enjoying whatever we get, we waste time in the hope of what we do not have, and in the greed of getting it, we lose even what we have.

Once my school's cricket team went out to play a tournament and lost all their matches. Their coach was hesitant to come to me. Finally, he said, Sir, our children who went to play cricket lost all the matches and they are scared to meet you.

I said, "Okay, send them inside."

When they came inside, I saw that everyone's faces were downcast. So, I congratulated them for the wonderful victory they achieved and said,

"Keep working hard like this, you will get success." Perhaps the teacher thought I was wrong.

He said, "Sir, they have lost all the matches and have not won."

I said, "That is why I am congratulating them on the victory."

The children thought I was being sarcastic and they felt insulted. Then I asked them some questions.

"Tell me, did you pay attention to your uniform when you left to play the match?"

"Was it torn jeans, weird clothes with the belt sticking out?"

"Did you spend time on the bus shouting or teasing each other?"

"Did you stay busy with your mobile phones till late at night instead of planning for your upcoming match?"

The answer to all these came in "yes". I continued.....

"After watching your mobile till 12:00 at night, were you able to sleep on time or did you wake up at 4:00 or 5:00 in the morning and go for your training?"

"Did you bathe on time, have breakfast, and practice on the net?"

"After every match, did you chalk out some strategies by watching the game of each of your players or the game of the players of the opposing team?"

Now the answer was "No."

Then I said, "Don't you think that whatever you did, the match was not at the center of all these activities? So, you practiced all those things which could have helped you in losing the match, if not winning it. So, you prepared for your defeat and you lost, so in this way you won, and you turned out successful."

And it is on record that next year the same team went out for matches and won the championship after defeating all their opponents.

So, if you say that you want to become a great player and believe in sleeping all day and not taking care of your health, it means you do not want to become a player, and if you do not become one, this way you are successful. If I say or ask someone whether Sachin Tendulkar is a great player, then probably everyone will say there is no doubt about it. But if I say that if he is pitted against a tennis player, will I again say that he is a good player? He can be a good cricket player because he has worked hard in this field and has practiced cricket continuously, which he did not do for tennis. The point here is that you should practice hard for what you want. Keep trying. And if you want something and don't practice for it. If you don't work hard, it means you don't want it. Then you don't get it. In that sense, you will be called successful. So, keep in mind that whenever an idea comes to your mind, make sure it is implemented in the real sense of the term.

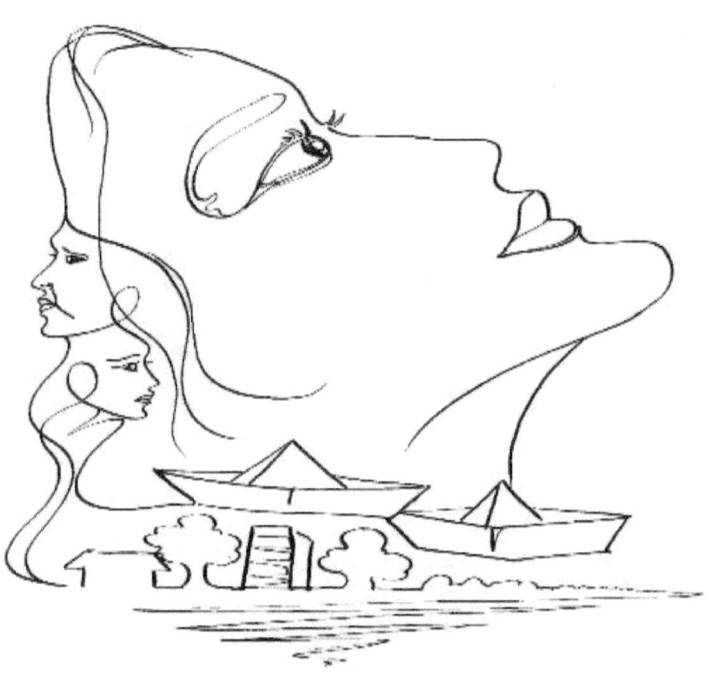

Moving is Becoming

All our thoughts and experiences—good or bad—are our own and for our own sake only. These cannot be given to anyone or taken away by anyone. Once it comes, it will not go anywhere. Even if someone else takes it, it does not mean it goes out of you or it is no longer yours. That thought is his only to the extent he takes it and comprehends it, or as much as you are able to explain it. You cannot explain all your thoughts to someone, and he will not comprehend them either. He will perceive only as much as he has prepared himself to perceive. Imposing your thoughts on someone is like not understanding the situation of others. It is not possible that the other person is also in the same situation and mindset in which you create your thoughts and summarize your experiences. Most of the time, the ideas we get are completely nourished by the events that have happened in the past. The past dominates you so much that you consider those events as a standard and give birth to an idea in response to them. These are the ideas whose authenticity has been ensured by yourself only.

You will find many saying that something bad happened to them in the past. They need to get over it or forget it. It has never happened that you have gotten over your past. It has become a part of your existence. The more you try to get out of it, the more you rush into it. Getting out is actually going inside. Outside and inside are relative to each other. The solution lies in just getting out without being aware that its you who is getting out of something. Do not think that you have gone outside from the inside because this thinking will bring the outside in as well. It is self-evident that you cannot escape your past, whatever it may be. Do not make the mistake of forgetting it, because forgetting is not deleting. Chances are that the reappearance of the stimulus will stir up those feelings in a much stronger way that may cause more harm than before. So, don't waste your time trying too much. Experience is experience. Good or bad is a decision that you take on the basis of inputs upfront, or it depends upon the circumstances. We make the mistake of considering it as a situation. Here we create confusion by mixing two different things. The situation is basically natural and is equally present for all mankind in equal quantum. It is our decision-making ability that transforms the circumstances into desired situations for the fulfillment of some specific purpose and divides it into good or bad on the basis of the result we get. So strengthen your ability and decision-making capacity, and do not try to forget or get over your past. This is just like adding yet another extra burden on you.

Sometimes you try to forget the past by focusing on something else or doing something new. This too is not advisable. It will be difficult for you to do anything new if the thought behind that is something to be forgotten. Is it mandatory that first you forget the past or get rid of it, then something new will happen? Is there a need to get rid of those experiences? There is no shortage of space in the mind. Let it be there only. Just like goods stored in a warehouse. It will rot one day without it being noticed. If you are an optimist, then believe that in the course of time, it will decompose and may create some favorable conditions for you. Now remember those old clothes of yours not currently being used are kept in your cupboard for years. One day, you feel happy by somehow throwing them out or giving them to someone. Just look at your refrigerator. You keep fresh leftover food every day and throw it away after two or three days, and heave a sigh of relief. On the first day, it would definitely be painful for you to throw it out. But after two or three days, the same activity gives you a joyful experience as it happens in response to the demand that comes naturally to save the rest of the fresh food from getting contaminated under its contact and to save your refrigerator from foul smell. In this way, imagine the anxiety of throwing away something that is no longer useful and the relief that follows. It was for your own happiness to make room for something new. It had to be thrown out, and you could do it.

This is not the case with thoughts and experiences. They do not occupy space. Therefore, it cannot be kept inside or outside in the same way. Neither does it have any form from which old thoughts have to be removed to make room for a new thought. It simply sticks to your behavior or personality and remains present till death or if you believe, in the next birth also in the form of samskara. Do not disturb it unnecessarily. Keeping it lying there may also help in sharpening your new thoughts continuously, though indirectly. The presence of green color does not mean that yellow becomes extinct. Green is simply dominant and yellow is recessive. The sooner we understand the role of these experiences or thoughts, the sooner and better our lives will be.

Time keeps on moving. Similarly, our thoughts and experiences too. Harmony between the two is life. This is where we lack coordination. One will go back again and again. Going back to the past is a normal process because it has been our familiar territory. It is our already happened state. Here we don't get any new challenges. There is no pressure at all to change ourselves. This is what we call our "comfort zone". For most people, they feel advantageous to have rest in their past, good or bad, again and again. The time spent here may not provide us with the necessary courage to fight new and unfamiliar situations. Here, spending more time than required is against the continuity principle of nature, which may lead to mental depression. This is bound to happen. Now you witness from very far behind, the time that has already moved so far forward, making it seem nearly impossible to bridge the gap so created. Here, I remember Newton's first law, which I had read in my childhood, that suddenly jumping from a moving train or suddenly applying brakes to a moving vehicle will push you either forward or backward.

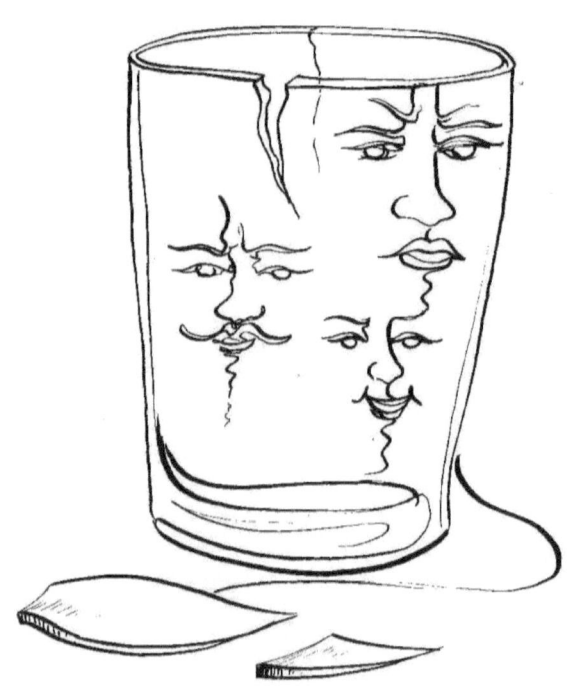

Break a Glass Everyday

Is responsibility or dedication required to carry out a job? When we do any work, we have faith in ourselves that we will be able to take responsibility for that work. Even after this, are we dedicated to that work? You may not be dedicated even after taking responsibility. Conversely, you can be dedicated even without taking responsibility. Are you able to understand this?

I remember an incident. I was posted in Northeast India. I used to live in the staff quarters. I was not married. I did not know how to cook. So I hired a domestic help to cook for me. My eating utensils were made of glass. I used to drink water in a tumbler made of thin glass. The day I hired the domestic help before leaving, she told me,

"Sir, please bring a tumbler made of steel in place of glass."

I was quite surprised. On the very first day, she dared to change my long-cherished habit.

I replied in surprise, "Why?"

She said, "Sir, these glasses are very thin and costly too. It can break anytime, and it will be very difficult to wash them safely."

I had become accustomed to having water in a thin glass tumbler. Then I don't know why I decided to give her a chance. Further, I wanted to see if she would be able to carry out this work responsibly.

I said, "Okay, I have seven glasses, you have to break one glass every day. All these glasses should be broken within a week. If you are unable to break even one glass in seven days, you will have to leave your job."

She found it very strange and perhaps even unwelcome. She must have considered it sarcasm.

From the next day onwards, she worked for seven consecutive days.

On the seventh day, I asked her, "Did you break all seven glasses?"

She said, "No, not even a single glass broke."

I said, "Now you are fired from your job."

As the conversation ended, she started leaving without saying a single word as if everything was ok for her.

Surprisingly, I asked her, "Why did this not happen?"

"Weren't you afraid of losing your job?"

"You didn't break even a single glass, you could have broken the glasses intentionally, at least to save your job."

I don't know what her state of mind would have been while doing the work. But I was able to extract some philosophy from here. It is possible that while doing the work, she would have understood the difference between responsibility and dedication. She must have thought that if a job is done with dedication, then the result of the work can change in her favor. Before this, she might have taken her work as a responsibility, but she could not have felt the sense of dedication. When I told her to break a glass every day, she may have become dedicated to her work. She may have wanted to see if she could actually break a glass. When the glass did not break on the first day while washing it, she may have developed the confidence that she can wash the glass without breaking it. She may not even be afraid that I will be angry if this happens.

She said, "Sir, if I am telling the truth, whenever I used to wash glasses, I lived a complete life."

It was an occasion to laugh out loud. How can someone say this, and that too with so much ease and respect, as if someone is making a polite request to break one's own valuable stuff, being too unconventional?

"The word 'breaking' kept me cautious. It provided a background that helped me to concentrate on my work."

"At last, it boosted my confidence that even if it breaks, I need not be worried. Where could have I got a more inspiring environment to work?"

"Here every day was an opportunity for me too, that "every day I have to save a glass from breakage." It's for you who think for me and also for that glass itself whose life was dependent on me."

"Should I worry about my job or live my life in such an independent atmosphere?"

"And yes, I have two small children and a husband too like these glasses."

It was a great learning experience for me. "Can living life and working for someone become that easy? Especially when both become one."

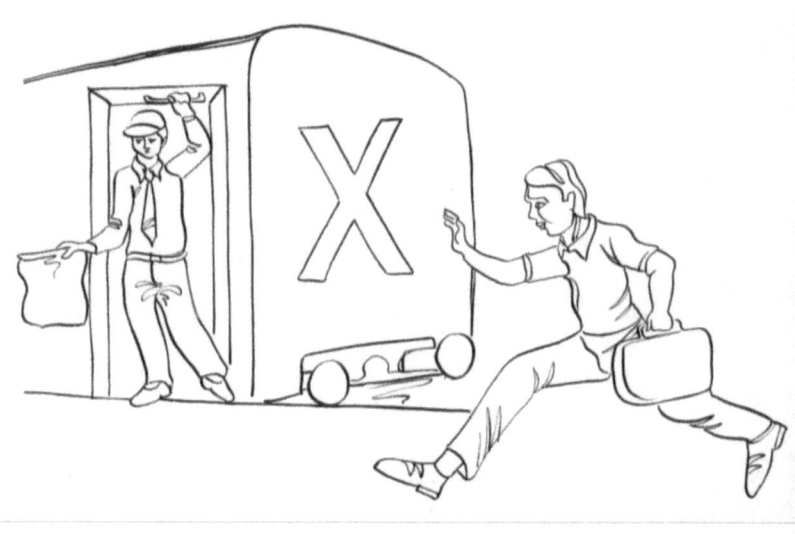

Problem: New Version of Old Solution

The problem invariably comes after the solution. There is only a whisper of the solution, which requires tremendous courage, concentration, and mental peace to hear the sound of its arrival. A problem is actually a new version of an old solution that comes with a lot of noise and hits us. For example, a lot of concentration and peace of mind are required to hear a sound of 20 decibels, but a sound of 100 decibels can wake up even a sleeping person. We usually get lost in our noisy lives and are unable to feel the initial presence of a solution. On average, it is hardly decoded by the common man. In due course, the same solution gets transformed and reappears before us with all the noise which is named as a problem.

This can be understood with an example. Not studying on time results in lesser marks, so one can think that if one had studied earlier, then one would not have to see this day today. It means you had a time earlier that you missed and got lesser marks. Let us take another example. I had to leave at 8:00 O'clock to catch the train scheduled to depart at 10:00 O'clock. I left at 9:00. As a result, the train got missed, and this is how the problem emerged before me. Then I thought, I wish I had left at 8:00. It means that if I had started at 8:00, I would not have missed the train. That is, the problem emerged at 10:00. But its solution was available to me at 8:00, which I did not utilize. You get angry. The situation is made worse. A problem arises, after some time you think that you get angry for no reason. It means, you had the opportunity earlier. You had the solution, but you did not take cognizance of the situation, and then the problem arose. Why does it happen that first, we should see the problem, and only then do we make ourselves ready to face it with all our might? It is also said that whenever there is a problem, do not react but respond as if the problem is not a situation but a power against which a separate discipline has to be created to deal with.

It is absolutely natural for this to happen. If we look at the process of human development, we find that struggle has been more important in human life than peace. From the very childhood, we have been told that life is a struggle. Problems will definitely come in life. If there is life, there will be problems. We have to move forward. Competitors have to be left behind. The more one struggles to move ahead, the more respect one will earn in society. The one who did not struggle did not live at all. Again, we already have principles like survival of the fittest or natural selection. In our social life, too, we have personified heroes and villains everywhere. In the beginning, villains are engaged in horrendous activities, and most of the time heroes have to fight for good and in the end after a lot of fighting hero prevails over the villain. So, it is necessary to postpone the solution until it transforms into a problem over time so that we can fight it, stay busy, and live our lives. As a result tendency to create problems emerges at every stage of life because we have to struggle. We have to fight. Fight for ourselves or fight for others. Then we have to invent such devices, which we can call ego, jealousy, anger, and greed which help in creating problems.

You mechanically doubt others. You start judging by your own eyes. The basic nature of human beings which used to be peace and cooperation, gets conditioned into arrogance and conflict. Now, even when you come forward to help others voluntarily, your self-interest will be sought in that too. Further, we have long cherished the notion that man is selfish by nature. Human beings cannot be trusted. This kind of conditioning has been taking place from the very beginning. Therefore, it should not be surprising if our nature has become like that. Now the question remains whether reverse conditioning is possible.

Nature never gets entangled in the dilemma of the problem-solution duo. This can be made even clearer from the previous example. If we had left at 8 o'clock or even 9 o'clock and had gotten the train, would we have been in this problem-solution conflict? Probably not, there would have been no discussion on the problem or solution. It means, both the problem and solution do not exist if you are tuned to time or nature. We accomplish a lot of tasks every day but problems may not arise during the completion of every task. It means it must have been completed on time, which is also natural. Therefore, neither we nor anyone else pays attention to it, nor is there any discussion or shouting. So, it will not come under the category of achievement. To achieve something, it is expected that first you see the problem or let the problem be shown to others. Those who want to achieve something have to understand or make others understand that life is a struggle so that they can be trained to create problems, and nurture them, but not to eliminate them. Those who are interested in living life or letting others live already know that life is a collaboration where problem-solution is just a timely tuned task.

The life of a great personality is similar to himself. If you listen to them they have a clear concept of the results rather than having a note on the problem or struggle. These people are a marginalized lot in their times till you listen to their followers or read their biography written by someone else, where you will see how much they have struggled in life.

Conflict and cooperation are two sides of the same coin but siding with a specific side has a different decisive impact on the approach or attitude towards life that can make life directional or directionless. So, if you feel that you are not capable of facing problems in life must understand that you do many things every day without facing any problems or achieve without an iota of struggle which in fact is the solution to the upcoming problem. You will be capable in the future also, just wait for the right time and space.

Again, there is unity in the universe. This unity is bound by rules. Our body system functions in harmony with natural principles in the auto mode of which we are not even aware of. It is the thinking mind that disturbs this equilibrium, and the system loses its balance, giving birth to problems at the atomic level. We naturally breathe. The digestive system, the blood circulation system, and the cellular system all work in coordination with nature. If we establish this kind of harmony with the nature we need not reach out to the problem.

Society was never created for blind race or cut-throat competition to move ahead in life. It was just to live a better life with the support of each other. There was never any intention to fight with nature. Rather, it was to cooperate with it. Even if you do not support it, nature will get support from you sooner or later.

Our birth cannot transcend the rules of nature and similarly, our death also maintains the balance of nature. When the control of our arrival in this world and departure from the world is in the hands of nature, then how can you be the referee of the game in between? And what about the mind, it cannot remain separate from the body, and when the body comes to its last, the mind cannot even save you. So, if in the end, you have to surrender yourself to nature, then why not comfortably merge with nature during your active life? Understand its rules, that is - timing, tuning, and coordination with effective regulatory mechanisms. Remember that every individual is assigned to perform supportive roles to keep the entire universe rolling in balance.

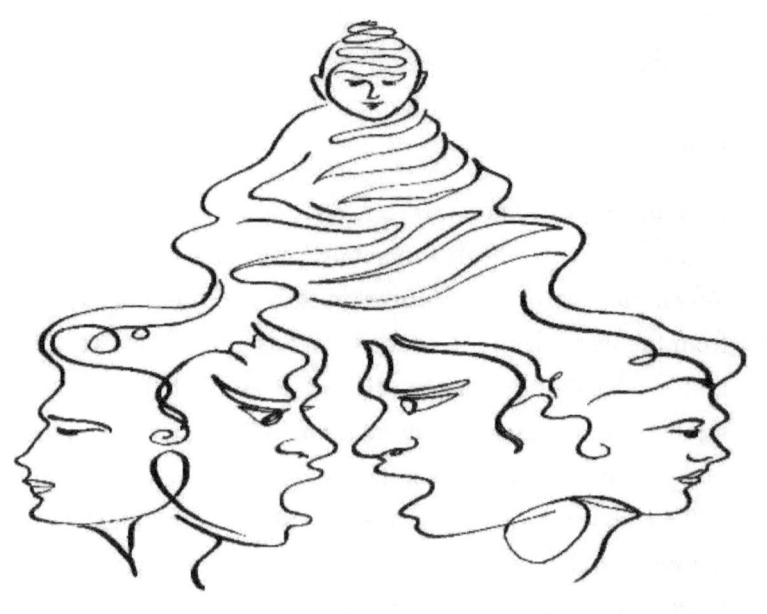

If Anger is Bound to come, Invest and Encash

We are often told not to get angry. Suppress anger. Do not allow anger to rise. Control it. Is anger such a state that should be given up? Do we really know the true nature of anger? If we look at anger as a viable option for a balanced lifestyle, its inevitability is a requirement of nature and an additional opportunity for enlightened individuals to choose from the given options. It is well known that the total amount of energy in the Universe is constant, but its form is absolutely temporary. It is dynamic and you can change its form whenever you want, provided your converter is working properly. Just like coal is burnt for steam and then electricity is produced from steam power through a turbine and generator attached to it. Similarly, with the energy obtained from anger, you can do wonders. You can even doubt the reality of anger, as without using it, we have also done greater things. Only that much energy has to be amassed from whatever source it may be. So, if you think anger is a reality and is bound to come, invest and encash it.

In fact, the whole world is a storehouse of energy. Every word that we speak is a literal form of power or energy. Every sentence spoken by us emits energy. You must have seen that people get excited by the speeches of leaders. Whereas the words of others may make you angry. On the other hand, the words of someone you love make you euphoric. When you listen to patriotic music or watch a movie, it generates the kind of energy that makes you thrilled. So, it is obvious that the speaker emits energy through the words they use and the listener receives the energy in the form of ideas or thoughts and, in response, the listener may give the energy back by clapping or cheering, and in return, the speaker again receives energy and feels excited. This is a cyclic process that invariably takes place in all types of conversation or communication. Here, it is important to see what kind of words you prefer to use. This selection determines the form and velocity of energy. Therefore, anger should be taken as a conceptual stage where the energy of the whole body is merged or fused. It may be compared to the energy concentrated in a hydrogen bomb. So its use should also be seen in this way. It means the energy of a hydrogen bomb can be used in human development or in its destruction. Today we have seen its use in both these areas.

Therefore, what we listen to and the kinds of words we choose while speaking affect us deeply. We are taught that we should keep company with good people so as to adopt their good demeanor. We may acquire these by observing their lifestyle. However, one of the main sources of adopting these behaviors is the conversation process. It is through the conversation process that we exhibit our behavior and also cause the transfer of energy from and to a person. Perhaps this is the reason why chanting 'Om' or pronouncing Ishwar/Allah/God gives us strength.

We have seen that the energy attained from conversation leads a person to get excited, fuming, thrilled, and brings a lot of similar consequences for them. All these outcomes have their own energy content that affects our mind and fuels it into action. Further, these energies have their own varieties. The most powerful of these is anger. When a person gets angry, he acquires the highest level of energy. In this state, he gathers all his energy at one point and ensures its outflow through conversation, usually through words. In anger, the entire energy of the body flows in one direction, due to which the energy required for intelligence, logic, and understanding the situation is not available.

This is the reason why an angry person becomes so powerful that he neither sees the time nor the situation nor his or others' circumstances. He just does what he wants. Actually, the basic reason for the origin of anger is our own weakness and the imbalance caused by the doubt of not being able to handle the situation within our own ability, and the wrong selection process. We should not take anger otherwise either. Animals have a natural tendency to protect themselves. Anger is just a defense mechanism of feeble and less confident people. Anger is the result of not being able to fight the circumstances and trying to hide and balance one's restlessness and nervousness. Notwithstanding everyone cannot be expected to be that strong. So how will the weak survive in this world? For them, anger is just a natural way of defense that keeps them balanced. For a person who is not enlightened or not knowledgeable enough and is unable to choose other options of energy naturally, this energy will be able to protect him from other dangers or balance him, even if only for a short period of time. Here lies its significance. However, the choice of guard can also be made in the form of being reasonably tolerant. But for this, you must be mentally settled at this level.

Being a classical physicist, we can see a self-restraint person like a convex mirror where the energy coming from one direction gets dispersed, thereby giving you enough time and energy to think of many other potential alternatives. In anger a person behaves like a concave mirror where the incoming energy gets converged or the energy gets concentrated, thereby giving you the wonderful strength to accomplish hitherto impossible tasks. Both are useful. At the first level, how can a person use his energy so that he can reach the highest point of life he wants to reach? Chanakya, insulted by Ghanananda, transformed the energy gained through anger into a great Maurya empire. There are countless such examples recorded in world history. Today, there are many great personalities in contemporary society who have made their best contribution by using this energy. So, here is a unique advice. Be an energy hunter-gatherer. Welcome the energy generated or expelled by others, demonstrated through rage and fury. Then regulate it and use it in different formats as needed and stay balanced. You can say that if anger is bound to come, invest, encash, and enjoy, only then will you be able to unravel its secrets.

On the other hand, when we remain calm, the energy gets dispersed. That is, we are able to muse upon other viable alternatives. Therefore, when there is a mishap, it is advisable to maintain patience so that we can consider various other options to get out of it. For example, large rivers where huge volumes of water flow very fast, causing deluge, can be regulated by building dams thereon, giving life to many development works from generating electricity to other welfare plans.

Now the question arises if you encounter an angry person, how can you use your energy and his energy? Here, there is not a confrontation or a conversation between two individuals but an exchange of energy is taking place. Just like if someone says 'well done' to us and we accept it, the energy of this word strengthens and encourages us even more. The better off will be the person who can store as much energy as possible in every situation, which can be used anytime in the future. Similarly, when we face an angry person, I am trying to give you several doable options-

1. If someone abuses us or gets angry at us, how do we react? We do not accept his abuse and return it in his own language. This will double his energy, and he will have the strength to abuse us even more, and we will not be able to use that energy either. Under the situation, the fight will seem to escalate because

both will be able to continue it with each other's energy. Then there comes a point when both get tired from exhausting their energy. There is little chance of any result, and after saying a sentence like "I will see you later", it is postponed for the infinite future. Relationships are bound to get spoiled, and it will keep you tense at least for some period of time.

2. If we accept his abuses and absorb the energy he provides us, we see that he slowly gets weakened. He loses all his control over himself. At some point in time, he succumbs to exhaustion. Use the anger energy released somewhere else and become stronger and sturdier.

3. If you allow this energy to rush inside and don't return it or use it elsewhere, this may annihilate you. Just like the energies, i.e. jealousy, hatred, distrust, and violence staying inside becomes the root of your destruction. This ensures the birth of the ego. The ego is a mental fat, which burns and emits energy of its own kind when you don't get what you want and things don't go your way. It is a nuclear furnace where a chain reaction or in-breeding keeps happening.

4. If you do not respond to an irate person at all, he will become angrier. If you smile even after that, he will become even angrier and may additionally show some kind of violence. There is definitely a reason

for this. Your calmness will disturb him. When a person is angry, he knows he is not in balance and expects you to respond to him equally so as to let him be balanced by seeing you imbalanced. You're being balanced or not responding will further leave him imbalanced. In simple language, it will be a challenge to his ego. So, he will once again attack you with all his might to bring you to his situation where he can now shout even louder. He may even resort to violence. Now you are free to defend yourself without losing your balance. But keep in mind you should not choose to use words that may give him back more energy. Let him get tired. Here you can make good use of the drop-down menu or switchboard theory explained in part II and III of this book.

Sometimes knowingly you have to show some anger to get work done. This is advisable too because in this case your health is not compromised. You only shout to make others be affected, leaving yourself unharmed. But it also takes some of your energy while you shout at. If you want to spend only a nominal amount of energy on anger and getting work done, you have a good option to choose. You just have to accept that you are angry. You may tell the other person politely "I am very angry, give me my money back." You actually tell your children often, "If you do not study now, I will become angry". You may sense this is very strange when I say that you should assume that you are angry. You will laugh, how can I assume that I am angry? Yes, exactly in the same way as you assume many superstitions and act scrupulously thereon. Exactly in the same way, when you assume that he must be thinking something bad about you and without any further investigation, you do remain jealous or hostile towards him for the rest of your life.

I would like to share with you a similar incident. The Wi-Fi at home was down for many days. Despite registering a complaint with customer care repeatedly, it was not paid heed to. Perhaps my request was too polite for them. They, too, might not have taken it seriously. Since I knew the adverse effect of being irate I decided to conserve my energy as I usually do. This time I called the customer care.

I requested him, "Before I advance my grievance, you please be apprised how I am going to talk to you."

A voice came from the other side, "Ok sir, tell me."

I told, "I will converse normally, but you must take it as I am angry. My tone, pitch, and frequency will be low but you have to multiply it by ten times more and louder." I continued…

"All this will be just like when you read the weather forecast on your mobile, extreme heat, 31 degrees Celsius, but feels like 40 degrees Celsius."

"Because I am really angry, but don't want to follow the anger protocol where shouting and harsh words are used.

This will keep you and me healthy and keep your respect intact too."

"If you agree, I should advance my complaint this way. Otherwise, should I do something that will make you feel I am out of my temper so that required pressure is put on you to find a quick solution?"

Believe me, as soon as I told this, I could hear her laughter. In this burst out, I could feel her level of wonderful commitment. This is how things can be done without challenging each other's respect.

Every time you have a choice, either you respond to anger with anger or respond to anger with composure. When you respond to anger with anger, you are wasting too much of your hard-earned energy. While spending money we tend to be misers as we know how difficult it is to earn money. It leads us to believe we should not spend it wastefully. But have you ever thought that behind earning this energy, the amount of time and money we have invested? So, its high time to work on your energy budget as well.

We have already seen that an angry person first gathers all his energy in one place. He not only gets this energy from the present but will go up to the past and the future to collect it. This is the person who had troubled me in the past, still troubling me and if not set right now or if I do not take revenge on him now, he will trouble me in the future also. By the way, this person had troubled my friends too. Now I can bang on him with greater force as the mass of anger energy will increase and so the momentum and impact will be. Now you can understand the enhancement of our gathering capacity to fuel our anger in this case. So, imagine the consequences if such an amount of contrasting energies to explode. Therefore, when there is a possibility of an explosion, at least one party should wait till the anger energy of anyone reaches its decay. At the same time, the anger energy should not overpower you. So, barring a few exceptions, try to support the energy of an angry person first.

That is, when you place yourself in front of a person with anger, first give your tacit approval to the points put forward by him so that he is not in a position to retaliate. We have already seen that in a state of anger, a person sans his logic, wisdom, and intellect, can do too many irritating things, and in most cases, after being exhausted, will regret it after a few moments. At the same time, he will feel satisfied that you listened to him. Now he will be in a position to listen to you too. Now only you will be able to present your side better and in your support.

This is about how to negotiate with an angry person unharmed. It is prudent that we should not get angry, but there are situations when we ourselves become victim of it. For example, you are standing in a long queue at the ticket window. Meanwhile, someone from the rear broke the line and blitzkrieg at number one at the ticket window. Now, no matter how calm you are, you will definitely get angry. Remember any such incident from your life. Can you stay in such a situation without getting angry? Whenever such an incident takes place, you will see that someone else in the line will certainly be in anger and he will take the responsibility to push him away from there. So in such a situation, you should stay calm and not increase your blood pressure. The other person will do your work.

If you believe me, anger is also a form of energy that is bound to be transformed at any moment. So it should be accepted that anger does not exist in its pure form, and it has no cause- -effect relationship with any event. This can be made clear with an example.

On one fine day, one of my employees came to my office and said, "Sorry Sir, I committed a mistake, yesterday I was carried away by the emotion that made me angry". I enquired whether you were made angry or if you brought anger with you. It means that when you say that you got angry under the influence of emotion, you mean, you are not responsible for this. Hence, you should not be punished for this. If something odd happens, we tend to avoid taking responsibility and in place put the responsibility on someone else. This is a completely natural response as we have been doing so from time immemorial, and its conditioning has become so strong that now we do not even know whether we have chosen anger as a response to any stimulus we face. Sometimes what happens is conscious activity, but it seems to have happened spontaneously. At least this much is certain that initially it must have occurred consciously and after a considerable period of time due to conditioning, it must have become the part of reflex action. Again, why don't you say that it was you who brought anger instead? This you will not do because you know that saying so would be tantamount to confessing that you are responsible and as a result, you deserve punishment. Isn't this a conscious activity? So the conditioning of not responding this way has also happened in humans long ago. If we observe carefully, there is no necessary cause-effect relationship between anger and the incident. Rather, it is a matter of choice. Suppose you get angry at someone for some reason at some time, then can you say that it is 2:00 o'clock now, it is lunchtime, I am going now, after having lunch and taking some rest, I will call you again at 4:00, then I will get angry. You cannot say this and neither can you come and get angry later. It is clear that anger has nothing to do with that incident; if it were so it could have happened even after 2 hours. So if you give some time to that situation then after 2 hours you can avoid its terrible consequences and can save yourself and your human relations.

Finally, I would like to give an important piece of advice. If possible, when you get angry, invest the energy inside you in a better option or maintain calmness and give others a chance. You will see that the person who has a grudge against you, will come and realize his mistake after a cooling period. And even if this does not happen, you will not suffer any loss in this situation because it is no longer a matter of your concern. At least do this with the person you love the most because relationships and very good relationships connect those dots of our lives that we cannot create on our own. This is similar to the fact that many life-saving nutrients cannot be produced by our bodies but are supplied by external sources. This is one of the many unblemished social messages given by nature, albeit indirectly and much silently.

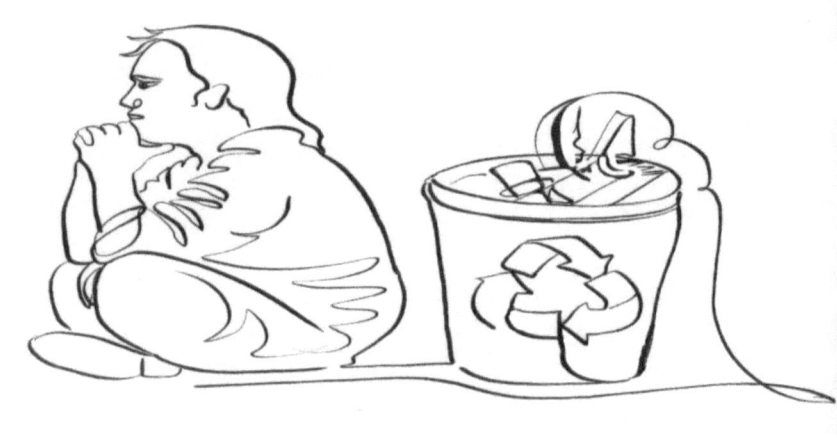

The More Nervous You Are, The More Scientific You Are

Here I would like to start with an incident that happened in my office. A day before this, I received a call from one of my employees late at night. He wanted permission to come a little late the next day. He said that he was feeling stressed due to working continuously for two-three days. As a result, his blood pressure had suddenly increased. It was not a question for me whether I should allow him to come a little late the next day. The question was, why do we arrive at such a situation? And with this question we started the conversation with him the next day.

Sir, "I have been involved in training educators for the last five days. A lot of preparation has to be done before this. In such a situation, I panic or get nervous."

I asked him, "Why do you panic?"

He said, "It is a habit, sir. Whenever any pressure comes on me, I succumb to stress."

I said, "Do you know how scientific you are? The one who takes the pressure or who reacts this way is more scientific. If I am not taking pressure, then I am artistic."

How do you panic whenever a task is assigned to you suddenly? This is directly related to the subject matter of science. Whenever we study matter, it is guided by two important principles of physics and chemistry. The main property of matter is that it wants to remain in its lowest energy state. Apart from this, through chemical bonding, atoms of a matter tends to achieve a stable electron configuration with eight electrons in their outermost cell to complete an octet. This allows it to remain inert. So, both theories state that matter is bound to be inert or inactive by nature. Since our body is also a matter, this theory naturally applies to our body as well.

On the contrary, the mind by nature always wants to remain active. This way we have given shelter to these two opposite forces in our lives. Matter, which is inert by nature, will never become active on its own. If it is in motion, it will remain in motion. It means it will have to work in both situations. Hence, for both these tasks, it has to take the help of an external force. This is endorsed by Newton's first law of motion or Law of Inertia. If we look at the nature of the mind, its very existence depends on its being in motion. It is ironic that these two units with opposite natures or qualities have to move together in balance. Now it is our duty to keep both of them in balance. Don't you think this is an art?

Let us try to comprehend their conflict in this way. In an ideal situation, both the mind and the body are ready to work. This is better reflected in those who are close to nature. As our brain develops, the imbalance between mind and body increases. If we look at the property of inertness, it means both the mind and the body don't want to work. Or the mind wants but the body doesn't. You will find a better balance in animals. Whatever they see, their body reacts to their immediate environment spontaneously. But since an intelligent human being can think more and better, we witness a relatively delayed bodily response. If we look at the workplace environment, some employees suddenly get nervous when the authority says that they have to do this work in two days. This nervousness is a natural device to bring the situation, arising out of the imbalance between mind and body, into balance. This is because whenever we have to do some work, the mind naturally gets ready first and much quickly, but the body's adorning quality of matter will not move.

If we are not in the habit of working for years, then the imbalance between mind and body will increase a lot. A stage will come when it becomes our ideal state, which we can name our "Comfort Zone", where the mind also starts adjusting to that, no more, no less. This is the reason that when a sudden assignment comes our way, we get shocked in the same way as if we follow Newton's first law of motion which states that an object at rest tends to stay at rest, unless acted upon by an external force .For example, when a bus suddenly starts ,passengers experience a backward jolt or when we jump out of a moving vehicle , we suffer its consequences .In the same way when all of a sudden we get an assignment we get panicky and stressed as the mind becomes active instantly but body remains inactive. You will also see that work done unwillingly will not give you the desired result and will tire you out more.

In this situation, the mind naturally exerts more and more pressure on the body. In response to this, the body too will also exert its strength to stabilize itself. The more the mind turns active to perform the task given, the more inactive the body tries to become. Now, to make the body active, the mind has to take the help of the hormone system that works under the control of the brain. It is a scientific fact that under certain conditions, endocrine glands make chemicals called hormones and release them directly into the bloodstream to help the body cope with various events and stresses. Its release provides energy to the targeted organs of the body, stimulating them to work beyond their normal capacity. Our organs work on the principle of "do or die". In this process, various organs of our body are adversely affected and gradually stop working. Many of our diseases, like high blood pressure or diabetes, are caused by the stress arising out of this imbalance.

Now this is not a story of mine or yours. This is an interaction between the mind and the body. We have to acknowledge that the mind and the body are two opposite extremes. We have to train both of them to work together in harmony right from the beginning of life till it ends. We certainly see people who become active as soon as they get work and this is their tool to maintain balance. You will find many older people saying, "I will become sick if I don't work". These are the ones whose mind and body work in harmony. We have to practice this unceasingly so that we get used to it before our mind says, let our body be stayed active. Such people are great planners.

In practice, we have found a unique pathway to balance the situation arising out of an imbalance between the mind and body of a particular individual. If my mind is very active and my body is inactive, then the mind demands an active body. So, now if I put my mind in someone else's body, I will feel lighter and balanced till my mind is engaged in taking rides of the other's body. That is why you criticize others unnecessarily, interfere in other's life, provoke someone without reason, and create doubts and discord between two people or groups. It will give you the impression that you have got somebody else's body to move along with the speed of your mind. You also feel happy if you make two people fight. Our mind becomes light, because it has found two or the maximum required bodies to get itself balanced. This is a virtual reality where we assume a virtual equilibrium to be true. There comes a time when it becomes too late for us to realize the truth. When the bodies of others come to their fall and you are unable to find the next, your mind will keep searching their refugee ad infinitum. It will not come back to its original and hitherto abandoned shelter. Or you never know it might have been repulsed by someone other's mind now enjoying the ride of your body that had come to fill the vacuum created by you yourself when you freed your mind to drive others. You have lost it once and for all. Now you rightly say that life has become lifeless, as with necessary exceptions, everybody's mind has found another's body to live in.

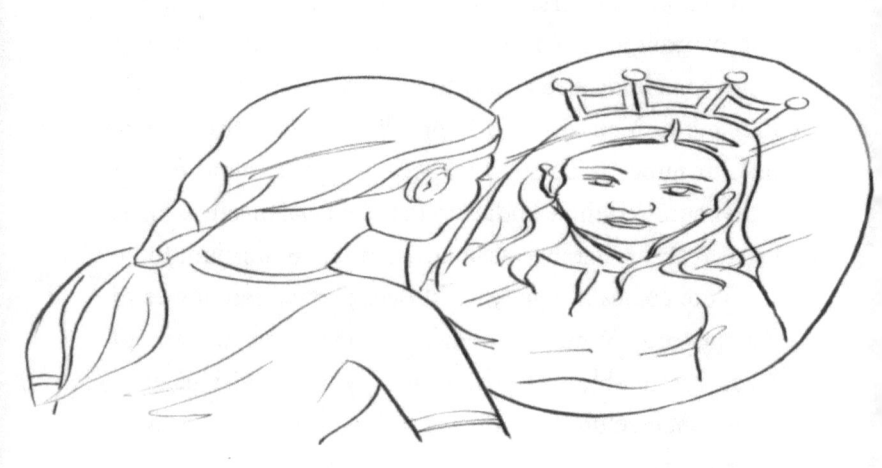

First Question: Leads you to lead......

In the true sense, we have to learn the art of living, for which communication plays a very important role. Self and other self are the most important elements in our day-to-day communication that decide the state and direction of our future life. Whenever we meet someone or someone meets us, it is of the utmost importance to know what the first question should be. It becomes even more important when we come across someone for the first time, in a specific time and space, or we meet someone once in a while, or meet someone after many days. It is very significant to know how our conversation should be.

If you think this is not that important, let me share an experience from my life. I was then the principal of a residential school. In every school, some children are good at studies, some children are not good at studies. If children are not good at studies, it does not mean that they are not good at any other activities. But there will definitely be some children who are not good at anything at the moment, who prefer to talk about issues which make them happy initially, but in the long run make their life miserable. So I did an experiment on the children belonging to the first and the last group. First, I alienated a group of children who were very good at their studies. They were docile, disciplined, and obedient. Then I made another group of children who were not good at studies and who had many other issues to talk about apart from studies.

These children lived in a hostel. Every Sunday, their parents or guardians used to visit them. I did a random sampling of some parents and gave them a questionnaire in which five questions 1,2,3,4,5 were written sequentially. The questions were:

1. How are your studies going on?

2. What kind of food do you get here?

3. Are you encouraged to play or not?

4. Do children bully you?

5. Do you get the freedom to go out?

I asked these parents to write down whichever of these questions they ask their child first and last while they visit the hostel to see their children. Apart from this, if they talk about anything else that can be an important question, then they may write it down. After getting their response, I prepared a list of those parents who asked the first question as to how their studies are going on. Again, I prepared a list of those parents who asked the first question as to whether their children get proper food or not.

When the response sheets of both groups of parents were analyzed the results were very surprising. The children whose parents or guardians asked the first question as to how are their studies going on, those children showed better awareness about discipline and studies and they did well in academics and other co-curricular activities. And the rest whose parents asked the first question about food or did not ask any question about studies, it was found that they were inclined towards many things other than studies and were quite serious about food.

It means, what did Sunday mean for the children? It was as if it were the day of an exam and they had to answer those questions whose question paper was already out. Now their strategy was to prepare for the whole week for the questions that were going to be asked by their parents. In other words, for a week a child was supposed to set aside everything so as to concentrate on eating so that he could tell his parents on which day the food was not good, on which date there was less salt in vegetables, on which day there was more sugar in tea, on which day the lentils were half cooked or on which day the food was very good. Those who knew that their parents would ask them how their studies were going, it was natural that they had to concentrate on their studies. So, what kind of takeaway from this exercise should we have?

Let's begin with the question that precedes the first question. Is there any association of the question with your life? In fact, your life, which is at the least, a combination of your thoughts, actions, or behaviour, is just like answering the questions you ask yourself throughout your life - to questions that you ask yourself or that are asked to you by others. When you ask questions to yourself, you develop a quest to seek answers for yourself, and when questions are asked by others, you search for them for theirs' benefit only. Even if you don't ask any questions, your life still exists in response to some question or the other. So whatever answer or the results you get in whatever situation you are, it has to be the result of your efforts or your commitment and courage to ask questions. Only difference is when your questions precede your action you are well aware of its upcoming results and have sufficient time and capacity to mold your action to your favour. If your action precedes the question, you must develop a habit of accepting whatever comes to your life, good or bad, as the will of the superpower, and now you can't do anything except repent for what you have done.

Therefore, you must be in the habit of asking questions using preceding WHs (what, why, how, when, and where) to yourself before embarking on any new task. It is like asking a child, What he wants to become? "What is the aim of your life?" is found to be the most sought after or most casually asked question in every home of ours. There is no surprise that he can say without thinking that he wants to become a doctor or an engineer, or an officer. In this way, the possibility of becoming something else will end forever. Thereafter, if you put a supplementary question, "How will this aim be achieved? There is always a big probability that it will go unanswered as if there were no such question at all. These WHs keep you alert and help you find the answer before the start of any work.

It is something like you are writing an examination in a school or college. If you answer a question correctly, you will get good marks. If you do not write correctly, you will not get marks. If you write garbage, it will definitely get you no marks but additionally, it will also irritate the examiner to the extent that the result may be disastrous for you.

A self-question can be asked by a student or by a teacher or by a patient or by a doctor or any person before going to school or hospital, or to their work place every day, "How will their time be spent there that day?" One can go for self-questioning every day in every situation. This habit keeps you aware and alive so that you can find yourself better equipped to deal with situations. It helps in making the next strategy and creates a favourable situation to achieve what you want to achieve. If you are a child and not mature enough to know the art of self-questioning, it is the duty of elders, parents and guardians to ask questions to them on their behalf, then the first question becomes very important in the life of the child who is on the way to become an upcoming contributor to the society.

Similarly, if you take an interest in answering others' questions, it will be helpful for others only. There is also a situation where you do not ask any questions to yourself by habit, yet you will keep getting results or answers. You should know the fact that if you have not asked questions for yourself, someone else must have asked these questions for you. Such a situation necessarily happens to those who make any of their action plans keeping in view how best they can show themselves to others. I am not saying that you should not listen to others or trust them. You simply convert the questions to make it for yours and at the same time equally good for others too, and be fully confident that it will lead you all to be smartly balanced.

The same thing applies to people working in the workplace or family or society, or various institutions. Different people live with different thoughts and perspectives, the basis of which is the importance given by them to why, what, when, and how.

If the child does not do well in school today, or we do not do well at our workplace, you will not get good results in the coming days. This happens only when you do not question yourself and keep doing things based on your natural instincts. This is what happens most often. You are only answering in the present, to the questions that you will ask yourself in the future. Today you do not study, your results are not good, and you will definitely think that if you had studied, your results would have been different. If it is so, the work done by you has been done in answer to the question that you will ask in the future. If your car meets with an accident today, there is a high possibility that you may have had the habit of driving recklessly. When this would have been happening over time and you would not have met with an accident, you would have never seriously questioned yourself that your car could also meet with an accident. Such thinking not only makes you careless but also keeps you away from the preparation to deal with the impending situations.

So, if the question is so important in your life, one can imagine how important the first question can be. *It can be said that the first question leads you to make your character and entire personality in due course of time, and the supplementary question gives you ample strength to see your desired personality confirmed.* If you get time, ponder on the time-based difference between some interrogative adverbs with compound interrogative sentences, the first part (before 'and') of which represents the present act and the later parts (after 'and') represent the past act.

What should I do, and what did I do?

Why should I do it or why shouldn't I do it, and why did I do it or why didn't I do it?

How to do it, and how could I do it, or how did it happen?

You will get the answer whether the question be asked much before the process of personality development or first keep doing to get your personality developed, only then you ask the questions. I may conclude that your grooming and consequent formation of your character and personality depends upon the type of questions you ask yourself all through your life.

Now, when we enter into any kind of conversation in our personal and social life, our first question is of utmost importance, not only for ourselves but also for understanding others. So, we should take care of how much attention we give to our first question. Further, on the basis of the other person's question, we can know what kind of person he is, under what situation he is in, and what kind of answer he needs, so that proper balance can be established. So, let me reiterate, if your child is unable to use the art of self-questioning, parents and guardians must ask questions to them on their behalf, then the first question becomes a leading question in the life of the child that will lead him to the point where he can be the effective contributor to the society.

Part-II

Balance

Law of Return

Parting, Knowing, and Returning

If we talk about science, we are all made up of the same elements from which this universe is made. The Big Bang event in the Universe released a huge amount of energy. The same energy in the course of time got mixed in different proportions, leading to the creation of this earth and its ecosystem. It means that the existence of all of us reduces the energy of the universe in the same proportion as the amount of energy we have absorbed. Therefore, we have to accept that we all are nothing but small packets of energy that have to move towards that supreme energy, naturally and inevitably, to make the energy cycle complete. We have been doing so knowingly or unknowingly. It is an eternal truth that "Parts emanate from the whole and later the whole attracts the parts and the parts themselves tend to end in the whole."

The Universe sustains its existence through three fundamental principles of Physics- Motion, Gravity, and Balance. In Indian philosophy, it is called Rajas (Movement), Tamas (Inertia), and Sattva (Harmony or Balance). These are the three forces that help the universe to manifest its aim and regulate everything in the world. Out of these three, Motion is the sole force that keeps the world alive. No motion means no life. That is why motion is found in the atoms of every object. If the cause of motion in matter is the electron revolving around it, then the cause of motion in the soul or consciousness is the mind. As long as these two are in motion, the universe can afford to maintain its existence, otherwise, all creation will come to a standstill. That is why its motion cannot be stopped, it can only be regulated. Regulation means there must have been some device that works as a brake and makes this regulation possible. This brake is Gravity. Both forces are responsible for keeping things in balance, which is the ultimate goal of each and every system. Be it religion, ethics, or behavioural science and what not.

What we call success or happiness can only be achieved by creating a balance between them. The balance we are talking about here is not a perfect balance, but a "near-perfect" balance. Perfect balance makes you inactive or inert and may throw you out of the cosmic system. If we talk about religious beliefs, salvation or Moksha can be considered an example of perfect balance. For the universe to exist, there must be at least some amount of imbalance so as to give the Motion, scope to move the object from a state of imbalance to a state of balance. This will help the entire universe to move. This I call a 'Smart balance'. A thin zone of near-perfect balance. Being a part of the universe, the rules that apply to the universe are applicable to us as well. In other words, our mind is a universe in miniature, and its expected movement is to merge into the universe one day.

This is the reason why we have always been anxious to know the law of nature. This would never have happened if we were not a part of it. If we have a desire to know our genealogy or society, or country, it is because we are a part of it. We can never have the desire to know everyone if we cannot identify ourselves with them. Not only this, the part is attracted towards the whole, but the whole also attracts its part towards itself in the same way. Just as parents have a natural inclination towards their children or have a longing to meet their children and their children also in turn keep longing to see their parents. Again, we can never decode the rules of the universe if that code is not a part of our mind. Our brain has been designed to catch the waves naturally, and a keen and ingenious mind can decode them. Scientists have done and are still doing something similar for us so that we can make our lives better by knowing the laws of nature as much as we can. This process is going on continuously and will be continued till the universe exists.

Knowing- Life is just a continuum of Balance and Imbalance

Life is just a continuum of balance and imbalance. Our life keeps on swinging between these two strings. We have been emphasizing gathering and using the maximum possible information to maintain balance among self, other selves, and the world and with the universe at both mental and physical planes.

When a child is in the mother's womb, it is a state of balance for him. Whatever movement he makes will be less conscious and more physical. As he comes into life, the laws of nature start applying to him. He will not have any decisions of his own. The problem starts when the thought process starts in children. The inanimate and non-livings that cannot make their own decisions are much closer to the laws of nature. Hence, it remains balanced spontaneously. As the mind or intelligence develops, it will try to establish its own separate and distinct existence with the idea of distancing and surpassing the other self, for which it will need different and its own kind of thoughts. The mind, which is like a physical electron by nature, provides a motion to an idea or thought. Once it gets a motion, it will remain in motion until some spiritual force acts on it. During this period, wherever the mind goes, it will generate its own thoughts, and the brain, which is a part of the body, will control the physical process accordingly with the help of neurotransmitters.

Whenever we talk about the rules of life, we have to remember that the self, other selves, animals, this world, and this universe are all parts of the same energy. They keep changing their form in the presence of various factors at different time intervals. We can say that there is a supreme energy bounded by rules, which has a certain purpose—to maintain the existence of the universe. But this supreme energy is distributed in different quantities in all of us. This is the reason why no one can be called perfect. Everyone has to live in harmony with each other. We tend to follow this also in our lives. Some people think that if they become a doctor or an engineer, they will achieve perfection and will be happy. Some people think that if they become more powerful than others, they will enjoy the happiness of heaven. Does this happen?

All the universal religions preach universal brotherhood. Unity is strength is a universal truth. What do these indicate? If our body is healthy, it is assumed that all the organs of our body are in balance with each other. This happens only when the thought process works according to this principle. We do not have the scope to go beyond the rules. Even a little amount of disturbance in the thought process will affect some or the other organs of our body. It leads to our physical discomfort or ailments. This situation will not be conducive to letting the healthy ideas grow. This cycle continues until our life comes to a final standstill. So, instead of controlling, regulating our thought processes in harmony with nature will keep us healthy. It is your first step towards what you want to be in life. Again, your own hard work is just a small part of the energy vis a vis the entire energy of the universe. That is why you will see that most people cannot achieve what they desire even after working very hard. They will need the energy of other people too. It is the most difficult task of life to make the energy of the people flow towards you. Here, the chances of advancement of those people increase who move ahead, taking everyone along. Here, your public behaviour and communication skills play a decisive role. Values like blessings of elders, love and care for younger ones, and attachment to plants and animals are expected here. The pathways of what you call success pass through this only. Even after all this, there is a need for coordination - with the aim and purpose of the universe, you can call it God or nature.

If there is even the slightest imbalance in the universe, it balances itself through natural disaster. When your aim or purpose matches with the structure or plan or design of the universe, only then you enjoy the so-called success. So, if you are to achieve what you desire, then your purpose, the purpose of proportionate people, and the purpose of the universe should all be in a straight line. Sometimes, even after working very hard, we do not get the desired result, then we say what mistake did we commit? There was no mistake, just your purpose did not match the design of the universe. When people say that if things do not happen as per your wish, it should be assumed that it is the will of God, who is the absolute administrator. We have to understand that individual balance has nothing to do with Universal balance. In other words, if an individual achieves what he desires, may be happy, but it does not mean he has attained a state of balance. So he will soon be replaced by another disposition. After a few days, he may not be that happy. He may feel disillusioned. The government also talks about the collective interest rather than an individual, and the interest of an individual may not match with collective interest. If we look into our daily routine, children feel that they are not being given junk food, they are prohibited from playing mobile games, and they are asked to study, but this is in their interest, which they do not know due to ignorance, but their parents or teachers know. Similarly, if our personal objectives do not match the objectives of the universe, we do not get the desired results and become imbalanced. To achieve a balance and desired success, we have to establish a balance step by step:

Balance of self with self i. e. balance between mind and body

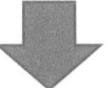

Balance of self with other self or other selves

Balance of self with the universe

This is the perfect order to achieve a universal balance and live a happy life. At the first level, only the self is involved. So, it is relatively easy to achieve. You can yourself maintain a balance between mind and body easily without being dependent on others. This can be achieved by establishing a balance between body and mind. This requires having a balanced diet, doing proportionate work and proper exercise guided by perfect thought.

Now we have to balance ourselves with others, which is comparatively more difficult because others are also products of their own circumstances and nourish their own kind of thoughts and may not be willing to yield to your pattern of thought. However, this can be achieved through the right thought process. Here behaviour and communication play an important role. At the most, you can achieve the balance at the first two levels.

But it is nearly impossible to achieve a balance with the universe. The reason is that we cannot comprehend the ultimate purpose of the universe. Only you can use your foresight or vision, carry out relentless effort in the right direction, and hold the patience of the highest level.

It is like trial and error or hit or miss. If it is a hit, we call it luck, and if it is a miss, we call it bad luck. However, it is only a linguistic atom. It is also prescribed in the Gita as 'Selfless action (Nishkam Karma).' Perform actions without attachments to their outcomes, focusing on the process rather than results. In simple words, do your work but do not desire the fruit. This also implies that you cannot say which work or which effort will help you to achieve your desired goal.

We can take the example of a circle-shaped hall that has caught fire. It has seven doors, and a man found himself trapped inside without knowing the number of doors latched from the outside. The resultant smoke makes everything hazy. Blindfolded going to the first door, but he finds that it is closed. The second one is also closed, and so is the third one. Lastly, he comes to the last seventh door which opens and he manages to escape. Here it could have happened that the person gets disappointed and loses the battle after finding the second or third doors do not open, but he does not lose hope and keeps trying, and finally, he finds the door that was open. You can call him a courageous and successful person who does not give up till the end.

It could also have happened that when the first door did not open, he could have taken a few steps back and reached directly to the seventh door so that he could come out more quickly unhurt. In that case, this person could be called a courageous and lucky person who does not give up till the end.

It could also have happened that if no door opened despite fighting hard, and he finally succumbed, that person could be called a courageous but unfortunate person who does not give up till the end but could not survive. This is how the cosmic order works because the end result depends upon the design of our ultimate administrator which is so inherently implicit in parts that always remains unexpressed or not manifested. This is why success can be personal, but spiritual happiness or peace never is.

To Return is to Join: Where and How?

Scientifically it's correct to say that every object moves at its subatomic level. At the same time, every object has a tendency to achieve stability or equilibrium. For this, the electrons revolving around the nucleus of its atom tend to form pairs in their outer cell in such a way that they attain octet. This way it becomes inert or balanced. So is the case with us humans also. Our mind also moves continuously in the same way so as to establish a balance by pairing with other minds having varied kinds of energy. These are natural and intrinsic qualities of human beings because every mind is incomplete until it meets the supreme mind. So, life is all about connecting. To whom to connect with, where, and how it can be is an individual process. So a person connecting with another person can be his initial step to achieve whatever he deserves. In this world, only he is successful who can connect with as many people as possible, at multiple levels. A leader winning the election, an actor becoming famous, or a person passing an interview endorses the veracity of the example given.

Similarly, pairing or connecting is a natural tendency of every human being. If a person respects others, he wants to be connected; if he loves, he wants to be connected, even if he fights or is jealous, he wants to be connected. Connection is natural, but forced and cultural disconnection or establishing a separate identity is self-imposed and self-directed. So you try to be connected consciously or unconsciously. At the same time, your mind tends to show how much you are different and distinct, and better than others. Here you misuse your freedom of will. So, in all situations, we want to be connected, but with the freedom of will thinking, why should I? He should connect or talk to me first. Why should I say sorry to him? Why should I greet him? Let him greet me first. Before he insults me, I should insult him. If the other person also thinks on the same line, you see the germination of jealousy, hatred, and quarrels as options for him to choose from. Then result will definitely be conflict and chaos. At the same time where there is an intent to connect from both sides, there will be a state of love, harmony, and balance. So, you have to decide whether you want to merge everyone in your mind by assuming yourself as the supreme mind and give rise to a conflict, or else by uniting yourself with others, you tend to move towards the supreme mind, where there is ultimate peace and ease.

Without accepting these principles, you cannot achieve success or even pass a competitive exam. The very meaning of an exam is to perform yourself according to the wishes of others. The day you connect with the minds of others or impress the interview board, you have passed the exam. You get a job, which may be the lowest level of thinking in one's life, but for a student who is looking for a job, it is life for him. For those who believe in religion, this supreme energy or ultimate soul or supreme mind is God. Those who believe in values can also find their meaning in this principle. If observed, this universe is full of energy, which is constantly in motion in the form of waves. Our mind tries to hook it through the process of thinking. This energy exists in a state of superposition or in every possible state. It is our mind that hooks it in a certain time or space to give it a specific shape. Our mind does this to keep in motion and activates the entire body. It is a subatomic state where only pure thought exists, neither positive nor negative.

In physics, there is the idea of a "black body". It is an idealized object that absorbs all electromagnetic radiation, regardless of frequency or angle of incidence, and interacts with and emits the radiation depending on its temperature. Our mind also works like a "black body". If we look at the energy content of our mind, it is very minuscule and limited. In the same quantity, it goes into the universe and freely merges with various kinds of energy moving in the entire universe outside of itself. So the significance of time and space increases a lot. You can imagine that there are infinite bundles of energy moving across the universe, and my own energy is free to merge with them. In fact, all of them are free to merge with one another. Then the combination of the energies comes in contact with the mind, giving rise to a specific thought, and the thought then gives rise to a clear and distinct physical response through neurotransmitters.

Just as the body gets energy from food, the mind, which is in itself an energy fetches its strength from its own motion. It naturally moves from high pressure to low pressure. Due to this energy imbalance or difference, the mind flows in a certain direction in a specific time and space. Anger, jealousy, happiness, fear, etc. are different combinations of this energy. These are available to us all the time as a choice. At this moment, energy is neither negative nor positive. All these are natural tools to bring us into balance. When these are used rationally, they often balance us. If these are used with reflexive actions (we call them emotions), they can disturb our balance, and ultimately, these choices are needed to balance us again.

For example, after the anger is over, we either apologize or forgive, or we get tired and calm down. It is also possible that after some time it gets transformed into some other form of energy. Keep in mind that energy always remains in a state of superposition, which our mind captures it in a certain time and space and it may transform into other states. For example, if I were to be angry at someone but couldn't, it means that I had let that energy go somewhere else or allowed other energy to fill the vacuum, or at the same moment that energy got mixed with some other energy. It is always advised that if you are about to be angry, you should start counting or else concentrate on something else. It is something like this. If I get angry at someone, and after two hours of verbal altercations, we agree to postpone it then can it be resumed after 2 hours? After fighting for fifteen minutes, it clocks at 1 pm. Can I say it is lunchtime now? Let's come again at 2:00 pm and fight. Hardly do we fight again. This is what is happening here.

We balance our energy from somewhere else. As Buddha said about the continuity of the world, everything is temporary. Nothing is permanent. We cannot bathe in the same river twice. This is the reason that if you wait, the energy of the required type will catch hold of you. On the contrary, if your mind is very eager to meet someone else and you want immediate results, your mind will catch hold of any kind of energy that might be going to some other place. In that case result will be contrary to what you thought. You will call it bad luck. Now, by habit, the responsibility of your haste falls on bad luck. It is like, you catch in the middle, a high voltage electric wire, going somewhere else and maybe to different transformers. It never means for you, but your inordinate impulsion coerces you to do that for which you pay the price by getting shocks. You wait for the bus or train until the vehicle to your destination arrives. It never happens, you board on whatever comes first, irrespective of the destination it goes. That is why it is said to wait, wait for the right time. If you plan on time, have patience, wait till the energy of equivalent strength or nature of the universe may pull you towards itself. Here it is important to say that you do not attract the energy of the universe towards you with your thoughts. Your energy content is very limited and negligible in comparison to the energy content and magnetic force of the universe. It is the energy of the universe that attracts your energy towards itself. That is why it is said to wait for the right time. Do not be in a hurry. This is the only way through which you can get what you call success. You can be instantly motivated by certain thoughts, like "what you think or contemplate repeatedly or manifest, or the more you commit to it, the more you attract the universe and you get, what you want from the universe." That would be enough to excite someone at a certain period of time especially when someone is under the grip of fear, urgency, and greed, and wants something big in no time and without doing hard work. In fact, it doesn't happen this way. Sometimes it may happen, and most of the time definitely not. You have the liberty to think that when you think repeatedly, the whole universe starts trying for you, what you can call manifestation. Thereafter, you have examples of few purposely selected celebrities who have achieved a lot in life by following this practice. But there may be millions and millions of people who follow this so called manifestation at the same time really work very hard, giving their entire lives to it, but they do not get what they deserve. If we take the example of the Olympic Games, there would be lakhs of athletes who nourish the dream of participating in such a great sports event, but does everyone get a chance to participate? This does not mean that he would not have dreamt it and worked hard. We should not doubt their level of commitment and practice. The universe does not have time or intent or any mechanism to give what everyone wants. The universe is not a matter of give and take but a matter of being in it or not being in it. If this happens and every person gets everything he wants, there will be nothing but chaos in the world. The scientific truth is that the magnetic field of the entire universe is much greater than our magnetic field in an individual capacity. You can say that if we do not follow the rules by which the universe runs, the universe will make you run according to its own laws. Can I think that I will live forever? To motivate again, we can say that the child who falls, learns to walk. This means that either the child or we know that he will learn only when he falls. This does not mean that you will learn only when you fall. The reason for your fall is not obeying the law of gravity of the earth and not being able to balance your body. Natural laws have never been discriminatory. For it, you follow its rules, you rule the roost.

Authority of Balance

Balance is the only absolute reality, and the principle of balance can be called a universal principle. It is manifested through the laws of nature. In the backdrop, it is supported by an ever-expanding universe with its entropic character, giving you more space to establish a balance. So balance acquires a centre stage of life, and life remains just a continuum of balance and imbalance. Only by adhering to this principle, both Purusha (Soul/mind) and Prakriti (Body/world/nature) can maintain their existence. The whole universe rests on this principle. If things are not in balance, they are active and moving towards achieving balance, and if things are balanced, they are still moving towards imbalance, endorsing the entropic character of the Universe. It is through this process the universe maintains its existence.

Every object has a tendency to achieve stability or balance which is the most comfortable position of anything. An object that is in motion is unbalanced and is a part of a system, while one that is balanced and inert is outside the system. It can again become a part of the system by losing its balance. This is what happens in our lives too. Whatever academic discipline we see today, they all talk about the cyclic and balancing nature of life. We can say, different academic subjects have been introduced to comprehend the extremely complex structure of life. All these insinuate towards one central authority- the authority of Balance. Just as Physics talks about energy balance, Chemistry has the Theory of the Octet. Biology has the content of metabolic cycle, life, and death, and free radicals. In History, we have a concept of rise and fall, and in Geography we talk about Isostasy. Economics stands for exchange and Balance of trade, whereas Sociology takes up the subject of social integration and disintegration.

These subjects reflect that all natural bodies and system try to stay in balance. Whether they are humans with two legs or animals with four legs or as many as they have. Whether they are terrestrial, aquatic or aerial, all move around in the world by maintaining balance. Whether we admit it or not, the principle of balance works on its own although we may not be aware of it, like biological process taking place inside our body, like the breathing process, blood circulation, and changing of sides of the body during sleep. Similarly, our behaviour is also adjusted to achieve mental balance. Whenever we interact with other people or groups, we balance ourselves. When we are idle or inert, neither thinking nor doing, we are in balance. As soon as any person or thought enters, our balance gets disturbed and we again move into achieving it.

Newton's third law of motion is in fact endorses the principles of balance. It proves that every action has an equal and opposite reaction. This is universally applicable to all objects or matter in the universe. The same principle applies to our body, also, because our body is made of matter. Whenever there is an action on the body from an external source, the body will also react so as to achieve the required balance. As far as the balance of the body is concerned, it acts or reacts like matter. It occupies space and forms an action-reaction relationship between two objects. Here you see displacement. As far as humans are concerned, apart from matter, it is also energy in the form of the mind. This may be the atomic state of the soul and responds like waves. Here, there will not be displacement like two objects, but there will be assimilation of two or more waves, the result of which will be the formation of different kinds of ideas. The speed, flow of energy, space, and time play an important role in the formation of ideas. The characteristic of thinking energy is to form any idea by merging with anyone, anywhere, anytime. Therefore, it is necessary to pay special attention, whenever external energy combines with your own energy and creates a disturbance, how will you balance your energy? This will have a direct impact on your mind-body balance.

Mind, in its primordial or atomic form, is a state of balance which can be called a state of peace in essence. It is a state of equilibrium where there is neither happiness nor sorrow but only a sense of being a spectator. This state is called salvation or Moksha in religions. But this is the only energy in our body that becomes active with the slightest of disturbance. Peace is its root, which is confirmed by the fact that, be it anger, hatred, laughter, fear, whatever it may be, peace will be seen in its extremes. Hence mind is meta energy that emerges from peace and ends in peace too.

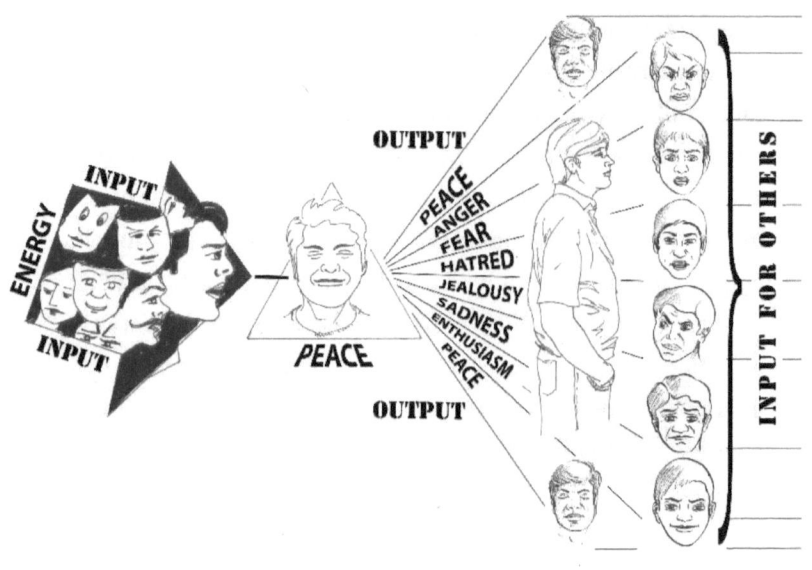

The Basic Nature of Life: Peace Dropdown Theory

The fundamental question is, whenever any action takes place in the mind, how will the mind balance itself? Here also nature comes as a savior. It has provided some mental tools, I call it M-Tools. You call these emotions. Actually these are not emotions but balancing tools generated from the rational brain –a garage where these are naturally preserved in the form of pure energy. Its different combinations can be used to make us cry or laugh or to generate anger or jealousy according to the situation. Every energy of its own kind exists in layers or in a continuum, where every next energy is slightly different and more vigorous or feeble from the previous one, depending upon its positioning, upper and lower down the order of the energy continuum.

Below are given examples of some such continuous chains of energy that we use these daily knowingly or unknowingly. Every energy combination has its own spectrum that starts in the state of peace and ends in the state of peace.

1. Spectrum of Anger:

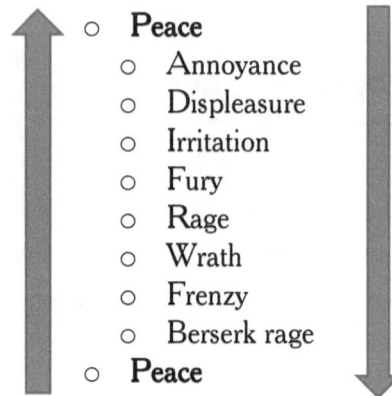

- **Peace**
  - Annoyance
  - Displeasure
  - Irritation
  - Fury
  - Rage
  - Wrath
  - Frenzy
  - Berserk rage
- **Peace**

Starting point of anger is undoubtedly peace. It's a fact, before getting angry, the person must have been in a state of peace. Thereafter, some potential thought makes one unbalanced, leading to a change from a state of peace to a state of anger. Nature and scope of anger change as its degree and intensity increase. The time taken for the reaction will decrease, more and more energy will come out. At its final stage, when the energy is completely exhausted, you will see, the person becomes calm and quiet. In our lexicon, different denoting words have been assigned for each stage of it, in order of increasing intensity of anger. It is just like the spectrum of colour in Optics (VIBGYOR), the subject matter of physics. Colors are arranged in ascending order of their wavelength and descending order of their frequency. Now, we are back to our own subject matter. If an incoming thought makes you a little unbalanced, we call you Annoyed. If its degree increases, we call it displeasure. If its degree increases further, we say that you are irritated. If it becomes more intense, we can say that you are in fury. Nature has fixed the upper and lower limits of everything in this world. So, a stage comes when anger also reaches its upper limit, passing through rage, wrath, frenzy, and berserk rage, which may be an extreme end of anger. When a person reaches this stage, he finds his energy completely exhausted and the mind becomes as calm as it was in the beginning. He may say – "Okay, what was to happen has happened. Whatever was inside has been vented out, now I am at peace." This way we come to a state of peace and divert our mind or get busy with some other work. So we have to understand that the series of anger is actually a journey from peace to peace. If you don't believe in this, you believe in otherwise ie once we are angry must remain angry for all the time to come. But it is not so. Even if you want to be angry, do so for all time to come. And if you think it is impossible to remain in anger throughout life then what is the rationale of being angry if you are to return to a state of peace ultimately? So, whenever you are angry, be mindful of which level of anger you are in and try to come back as soon as possible otherwise you will definitely be back to a state of peace but only after spoiling your health and the relationships and sacrificing your priorities in life.

2. Spectrum of Fear:

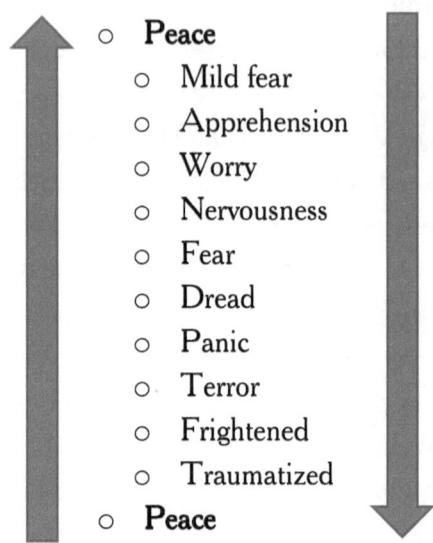

- **Peace**
  - Mild fear
  - Apprehension
  - Worry
  - Nervousness
  - Fear
  - Dread
  - Panic
  - Terror
  - Frightened
  - Traumatized
- **Peace**

On the same pattern, we now see a continuous series of fears. Before the fear strikes, you must have been in a state of peace. Meanwhile, a scary thought might make you unbalanced, leading to a change of state from a state of peace to a state of fear. As its degree increases, the intensity of fear increases, and accordingly, the different denoting words are assigned to each state. The continuum or series of fear travels from mild fear to the maximum level of fear. Depending on its intensity, fear energy starts from mild fear, which is a slight feeling of unease or concern. In between, we have different stages of fear energy in ascending order. Mild fear is followed by apprehension which means worry about something that may happen. The next stage is being worried, which is an ongoing feeling of anxiety about possible problems. Next comes nervousness, which is a state of being tense or uneasy, followed by fear, a strong apprehension, caused by perceived danger or threat. Next in order of increased intensity is dread, an intense fear about a future event. Panic is a sudden, overwhelming fear leading to irrational behavior. Terror **is** an extreme fear that paralyzes or overwhelms. Frightened, a state of being suddenly afraid or alarmed, ends in a traumatized state where we have severe disturbance caused by intense fear or shock. At this stage, we are so scared that we become fearless to the extent that we do not feel even a little bit of being afraid. It means the energy of fear is completely exhausted, and the mind becomes calm. You say – "okay, what was to happen has happened, now whatever happens I will see." This way we come to a state of peace. So we have to understand that the chain of fear is actually a journey from peace to peace.

Fear does not mean that you get scared. Your fear is also a tool to balance yourself. If you do not choose it at the first available opportunity, you will see that the mind will use other parts of the body to find a balance that can have an adverse effect on your body. Like, if you suddenly see a snake in the dark, the sound of "Aah" will automatically come out of your mouth. This reaction balances you. If "aah" does not come out, you will notice that your heart will start beating at a much faster rate. So choose the first and easiest option you have and stay safe.

3. Spectrum of Hatred:

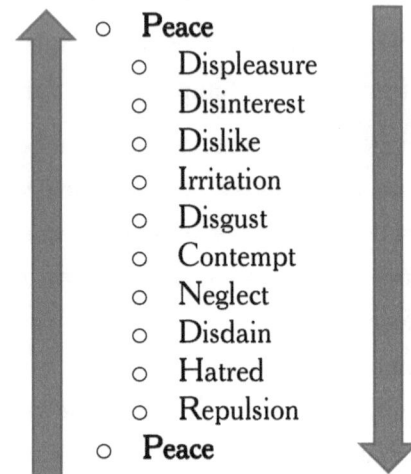

- **Peace**
  - Displeasure
  - Disinterest
  - Dislike
  - Irritation
  - Disgust
  - Contempt
  - Neglect
  - Disdain
  - Hatred
  - Repulsion
- **Peace**

Similarly, if we go on the chain of hatred before hatred originates, the person must have been in a state of peace. From the state of peace, there is a slight imbalance, we get into a state of displeasure. When we don't stop here, we develop a disinterest, which is a lack of interest or enthusiasm for something. Thereafter, in ascending order of intensity of hatred, we have dislike, a mild disagreement, or aversion. Irritation is a slight feeling of annoyance or anger. Disgust, is a feeling of aversion or repulsion. Contempt, considering someone to be inferior or worthless. Neglect, intentionally ignoring or overlooking. Disdain, a complete lack of respect. Hatred, is an intense feeling of aversion and opposition. Repulsion is a strong feeling of hatred, which is the upper limit of hatred, and finally, due to extreme hatred, we are unable to compete or fight further and become calm.

It can be supported by the example of Mr. X. His neighbor's child passed the exam in the first division in his class. His father Mr. Y distributed sweets in his society as a mark to show his achievement and resultant happiness. Since Mr. X's socio-economic status was almost the same as that of Mr. Y, and his child was also studying in the same class, but his result was not that good, Mr. X's balance was disturbed. In the next few days, some more good things happen to Mr. Y. His respect increases in the neighborhood, which makes Mr. X feel that he cannot do better than him, due to which he becomes more unbalanced and in order to regain his balance, he starts showing displeasure, disinterest and develops a disliking towards him and blaming his fate. A few days later, Mr. Y gifted his child a motorcycle on his birthday. Now his balance is further disturbed because his financial position does not allow him to give a motorcycle to his own child. In response to this, Mr. X tries to keep himself in balance by developing a feeling of disgust, contempt, and neglect towards Mr.Y, saying that Mr.Y is spoiling his child by giving him a motorcycle at such a tender age. Further, Mr. Y's status was on the rise day by day. In response, Mr. X develops a sense of disdain and hatred and starts despising, insulting, or mocking him even in public places. His balance is completely disturbed when Mr. Y lays the foundation of his new house. It means Mr. X reaches a level of hatred or resentment or repulsion from where it is no longer possible to compete, react, or respond to him. Now Mr. X feels he can no longer compete with Mr. Y. This is not the story of Mr. X and Mr. Y. It is very common in our day-to-day life. If it is your story, how do you keep yourself in balance? Either you join him by saying Mr. Y has achieved this position through all his hard work, and we all should take inspiration from him, or else you break your connection with him once and for all – "What difference does it make to me, I have to look after myself only". Now you are calm and focus your attention somewhere else. So, your hatred energy starts from peace and ends in peace. So don't go too far, crossing the limit of peace, otherwise you will pay double the price for to and fro journey.

4. Spectrum of Jealousy:

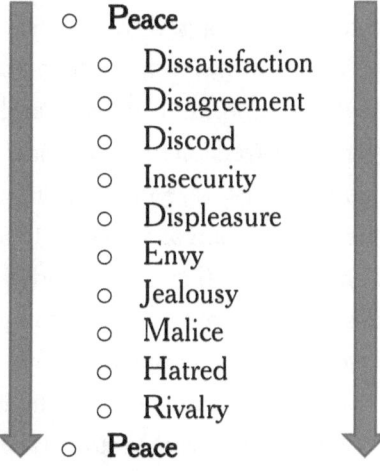

- **Peace**
  - Dissatisfaction
  - Disagreement
  - Discord
  - Insecurity
  - Displeasure
  - Envy
  - Jealousy
  - Malice
  - Hatred
  - Rivalry
- **Peace**

On the same pattern, we now see a continuous chain of jealousy. Before we develop a feeling of being jealous we must have definitely been in a state of peace. Varied types of thoughts, challenging our status quo and our inability to negotiate the situation, at the moment, may unbalance us. This hastens change from a state of peace to a state of jealousy. As its degree increases, the intensity of jealousy increases. Each situation has been assigned different denoting words. The continuum or chain of jealousy goes from dissatisfaction to rivalry. Process starts from dissatisfaction, which means a feeling of not being content. The next stage is the disagreement which means a lack of alignment in thoughts or feelings, then discord brings a mild conflict or dispute with someone and insecurity, generating a feeling of doubt or apprehension about one's status or importance, whereas, displeasure ignites feelings of unhappiness or discontentment. This is followed by envy, which produces mild resentment. Thereafter, we enter into jealousy that gives a feeling caused by someone else's goodness or success. Malice brings a deep feeling of hatred and opposition toward someone, and hatred stands for an intense feeling of rejection or aversion towards someone. The string of jealousy ends in rivalry, carrying a strong desire to surpass or outdo someone. As soon as we come to a state of rivalry, we try to continue with it, till we go ahead of them or they go far ahead of us where we are unable to compete with them. By that time, we realize we have wasted our valuable time and resources, causing irreparable damage to ourselves. Here, the energy of jealousy goes into oblivion and submerges into calmness. We may say - let's start afresh and get back to business." This way we come to a state of peace. So, we have to understand that the chain of jealousy is actually a journey from peace to peace.

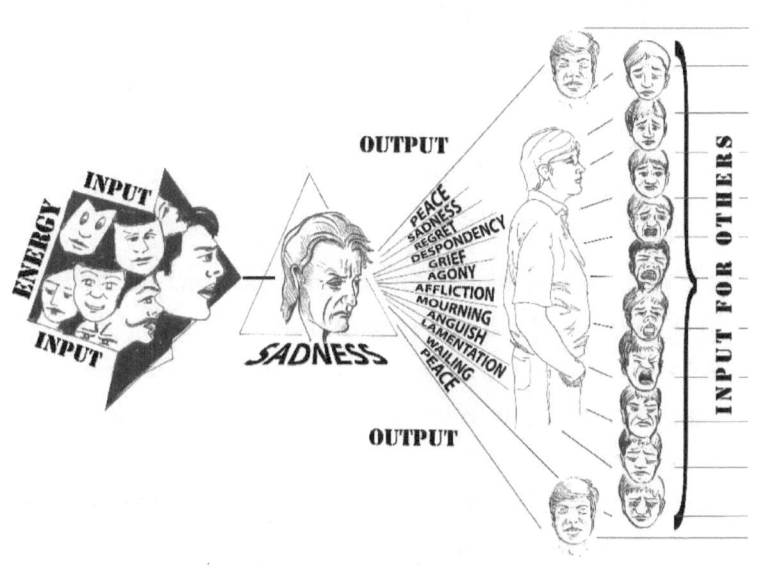

5. Spectrum of Grief/Sadness

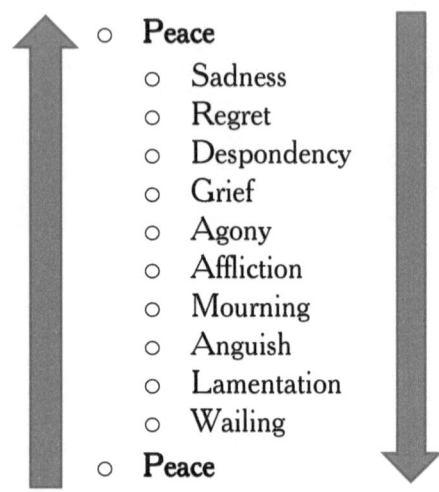

- **Peace**
  - Sadness
  - Regret
  - Despondency
  - Grief
  - Agony
  - Affliction
  - Mourning
  - Anguish
  - Lamentation
  - Wailing
- **Peace**

Now, look at the continuous chain of grief or sadness. You must have been in a state of peace before entering into a state of sadness. As soon as you get to know something happens contrary to your expectations, or as a student, you score fewer marks in the examination or are unable to secure a place in a competitive examination, even after doing all the hard work, you become unbalanced to the extent the event disturbs you. If the degree of grief is less, you just become sad and balance yourself immediately by uttering simply "OH". If the degree of grief increases, you regret, which means a feeling of remorse or sorrow. Next in order will be despondency, a state of deep mental depression or hopelessness. Next in order is grief, a feeling of pain caused by loss. Agony is deep anguish caused by an event or situation. Affliction is a state of intense suffering, often with self-reproach. Mourning, deep sorrow due to the death or loss of a loved one. Anguish, a strong feeling of sorrow combined with anger. Lamentation, expressing intense grief by crying out loudly. Wailing, is an expression of widespread and intense sorrow, and finally, at this level, we can balance ourselves either by shedding tears or by going into depression, we become absolutely calm. Another mature balancing act is believing that 'everything will be fine with time'. Now, we can think whatever happened has happened. It was God's will. You now resume your work as usual.

6. Spectrum of Enthusiasm/Happiness

As far as enthusiasm or happiness is concerned, does it also unbalance a person? The question is definitely a queer one – everyone feels that happiness is not a state of disturbance but a kind of satisfaction. But you will be surprised to know that enthusiasm or happiness unbalances us in the same way as grief or anger or hatred does. Putting it in a situation - You have topped in a competitive exam or achieved something which is rare for you and a matter of great happiness for your family. You are away from your family. How much time do you take to inform them? The greater the achievement, the less time you will take to share it with your family members. What is it? That great achievement makes you so unbalanced that whether you are unwell or in a state where you cannot stand up, you will run and inform your family immediately, or you will use your mobile phone in no time to get the information shared. The moment you share your excitement with your parents, you become balanced, but this disturbs the balance of your parents now. That's why only then they too can react happily and balance themselves by saying "Well done" or "Congrats". Does it ever happen that your father says "Humm" and leaves? His only saying "Humm" will further unbalance you.

If you are elated or excited, you balance yourself by hugging someone you love. This is often seen in the playground. Under the seize of exuberance and cheerfulness, especially when a player scores a goal in a football/hockey or takes a wicket in cricket or when they basket the ball in basketball, everyone runs, hugging and even jumping on each other. They have no fear that someone's bones or ribs may break or even they can hurt themselves. You can understand what I am saying. So, this kind of reaction is natural to balance the imbalanced state of mind caused by contentment, happiness, joy, or excitement. So, here also we find the spectrum of happiness:

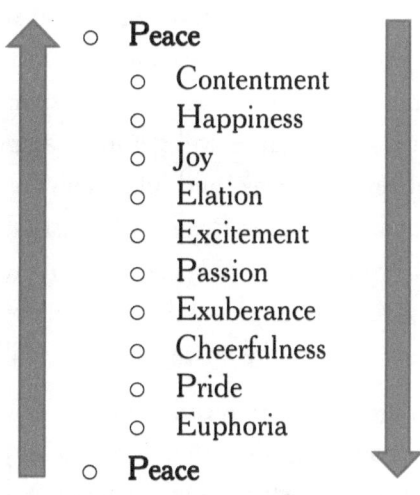

- **Peace**
  - Contentment
  - Happiness
  - Joy
  - Elation
  - Excitement
  - Passion
  - Exuberance
  - Cheerfulness
  - Pride
  - Euphoria
- **Peace**

When we see a continuous series of enthusiasm, we find that before excitement or happiness takes place, a person must be in a state of peace. The moment he receives good news or favorable results leaves himself in a state of imbalance. In ascending order, they can feel contented, a feeling of satisfaction with a situation or achievement. Happiness, a general and pleasing mental state. Joy, a deep and pleasant feeling of delight. Elation is a state filled with cheerfulness and joy. Excitement, a mood full of new energy and enthusiasm. Passion is an intense enthusiasm or motivation for a task. Exuberance is a feeling of great joy. Cheerfulness is an experience of extreme happiness and satisfaction. Pride, a feeling of honor or self-esteem resulting from an achievement, ultimately ends in euphoria, an intense state of happiness or excitement where one loses control.

So, all need to be balanced. We normally express these imbalances through our body posture and body language like, smiling, a comfortable body posture, an excited state of body, pleasant way of speaking. As its intensity increases, each level gets a name as written above. In response, to ensure balance, our body language will get more aggressive and finally, it reaches the peak and ultimately rests in calmness. The immediate euphoria caused by just winning the World Cup or Olympic medal in sports gets balanced by aggressive body language, but after two days, they all become calm and they all now wait for the next match peacefully.

These examples are of all the possible mental states we are normally in. Basically, our ideal state is a state of peace. This state remains as long as external energy does not disturb the ideal state. This state depends on the amount of energy we exchange and in what combination. In simple terms, whenever we think or talk to someone, we are emitting or receiving waves, we can call this condition as wave disturbances, leading to the formation of different thought patterns either to balance out the things or disturb the disturbances further. These thought patterns are found in the form of a continuum of energy, which we can choose at our discretion. Each form of response that we can choose from the M-Tools, has its own spectrum, in turn, it has its own level of intensity and impact. It is only to comprehend this spectrum in a simpler way, I have put it in an ascending order depending on its intensity, or the quantum of energy it absorbs, and the quantum of energy it releases. This also determines its momentum and impact on the body and mind of a human being. But it doesn't mean a person will travel down in the same hierarchical order. One can find oneself at any level, or one can start from the third stage and jump to the seventh stage, or from anywhere to anywhere up or down the order. All depend upon the intensity of disturbance they receive from outside. But, in all cases you feel the peace in the end. For example, we can respond to anger with the help of any level of fear or hatred or grief, or smile, or otherwise.

It is worth pondering why we should respond to anger with anger or hatred with hatred, especially when we know that it is only a question of maintaining balance and we have simpler options. If I am to be believed, this task is as easy as picking out fruits or vegetables from the vendor or recognizing your child in a crowd. What we call emotions today is actually just a bundle of energy and conscious choices to balance ourselves. The more mature a person is, his choice will be more mature. For example, if someone gets angry with us, we have many tools available from the drop-down menu, like laughing, remaining calm, being afraid, hating, etc. Hence, from now onwards, if you get angry, choose the safe option. If not immediately, after a few hours, you are going to feel wonderfully good. This is the master stroke to achieve success in all walks of life.

Principle of Balance

Some Stories from My Life

All these stories are part of my life, provided a rare learning on how do we transform our energy in our day to day life through reasoning, discretion and intellect through involvement of mind. I was a principal of a school then, I once received a complaint from a parent that a teacher had scolded his son badly.

To find out the truth, I called that teacher and asked him, "Is it true?"

The teacher admitted, "Yes, Sir."

I asked, "Why did you do that?"

The teacher said, "He does not study, so I scolded him."

I asked in reply, "The child must have started studying after your scolding?"

The teacher replied, "No, sir. He is so stubborn, not listening to anyone. I have been scolding him for many days but to no avail."

I asked, "If he did not listen even after you scolded him once, what was the justification for scolding him again?"

I can understand that every teacher in the world who feels that their student is not studying is bound to get stressed.

Being stressed means that you are not in balance. To achieve this, you can get angry, scold someone, or make him understand with love and care. It is better to choose such an option from the drop down menu, mentioned in this chapter, to regain your balance, and at the same time take care of whether the other person is also able to balance himself thereafter. In this example, the teacher chose the option of scolding the child, by which he restored his balance and became inactive. But, this made the child unbalanced.

Here, it is also important to see that the basis of continuity in the process of scolding may not be non-studying habit of the child but the teacher would have definitely been unbalanced by the fact that the child did not listen to him even after telling him several times. The teacher's continuous disregard would have made the teacher unbalanced. To balance himself, the teacher, following the drop down theory, chose the option of scolding. Now the teacher got himself balanced and moved out of the frame. Now it is worth seeing how the child, who is unbalanced after being scolded, will balance himself further. So basically, here it was a battle of balance.

Now, what happened, the teacher regained his balance, but the child who was rebuked, lost his balance. Now the child had many options to regain his balance. Like, he could have cried, not reacted at all, gotten violent, or he could have told his parents. He chose the last option. As he told his father, the child regained his balance, but the father lost his balance. Now to restore his balance, he complained to the principal and regained his balance. Now the principal felt disturbed and called the same teacher. To regain his balance he reprimanded him and regained his balance. The teacher was hurt by the reprimand of the principal and he lost his balance again. To regain his balance, this time he did not choose the option of anger but a safe and easy option - to apologize and promise not to do this in the future. Here, the teacher's assurance of not repeating such a mistake in the future balanced the principal, and the principal forgave him. This means that in both incidents the teacher's balance got disturbed, and in both cases the teacher applied his mind and chose different options at two different times to balance himself. Because by getting angry at the children he felt that the children could not harm him, and by getting angry with the principal he could harm himself. Thus, the cycle is complete. It would have been a different matter if the teacher had not apologized and the principal had also not forgiven, then this cycle would have continued further. Sometimes this cycle is completed only after life ends.

It means, in order to keep oneself balanced in a practical way, a person chooses the options by application of mind according to the situation and his ability to deal with it. These options are chosen in such a natural way that the person does not even know how it is happening. He just feels he is doing this in reaction to the immediate incident.

Now, I am putting here some other form of energy, not explained so far due to the paucity of space. These are laughter, surprise, and crying. These have their own continuum or spectrum and are used by us to respond the external stimuli or disturbance so that the required balance is achieved. It means that whenever any ideas or thoughts enter into the mind of a person from an external source, in whatever amount, it disturbs his balance in the same amount. Accordingly there will be a reaction in the same amount to regain the balance. For example, if someone cracks a joke, you go along the spectrum of laughter and you see, you laugh as much as the joke disturbs you. You cannot laugh hysterically at every joke or cry out loud at every mishap. Your reaction depends on how much your balance is disturbed. So, if it's a power of joke that makes you laugh, then, in response, everyone will laugh in equal amounts and in the same way, but it is not so.

Every person will have a different reaction to the same joke. Like, not laughing at all, only moving the lips, smiling slightly, laughing by showing the teeth, laughing by separating the lips, laughing from the throat, laughing loudly, or laughing by rolling on the ground or even getting angry. All these reactions must be in response to regaining the amount of balance lost while listening to the joke. Similarly, the word "Oh" is uttered after seeing some surprising things. Screaming after seeing a scary thing is an incident of balancing oneself after getting unbalanced by all external threats or events. When you suffer a big loss, you cry, but crying also has its own extreme, where you become absolutely silent after crossing its upper limit. The fact is that sometimes a person reaches such a state of shock that he does not even shed tears. In such a situation, so that the person does not lose his balance and become unconscious or otherwise, an attempt is made to make him cry so that he can regain balance.

People who do not know this fact always consider crying in the wrong way, as if crying is undesirable. Many times, we see that a crying person is advised to laugh forcibly. We have to understand that the person who is crying is trying to balance himself, and since the other person is not crying, he feels laughing is the right thing to do.

It is often seen that people in higher positions want to control their subordinates by controlling their natural reactions. You, as head of your office, want to laugh at the jokes of your subordinates, but will not laugh. You feel that your laughter will reduce your control over the employees. This method is adopted to balance your desire for power. But, this is not good for your mental balance. Hence, it is advisable that if you cannot laugh openly, you should at least laugh in a light-hearted manner. Again, if it really isn't worth it, you should, at least, you can say something about the jokes, cracked, otherwise the balance of your employees will be disturbed, as nobody wants to be going unnoticed, especially if it happens in the presence of other colleagues. In response, he will lose his trust and respect in you. And, he will balance himself by not working for you wholeheartedly. By doing this, he will be able to maintain balance among his colleagues, otherwise, he will have to face taunts.

Hence, I should say that the unnatural balance created by these people creates the possibility of so-called, emotional disturbance. This hinders the attainment of the objectives of the organization. Experience shows that productivity is higher in a system where interpersonal relations move towards establishing a balance rather than disturbing it. This kind of disturbance may produce immediate results, but it cannot be maintained for a long time. It would be appropriate to say that even a perfect balance will render our system inactive. Hence, reasonable imbalance is desirable for the development of an institution or a system. The important thing is that the aim should be to achieve a workable balance and not to establish a perfect balance. This can be done through smart balancing. Here, inter-personal relations should be regulated effectively, keeping in view to ensure balance at both ends.

I remember an incident. In the institute where I used to work, there was a management head who was very knowledgeable, but he also wanted others to get this recognized. Here I want to place the fact that it was not the era of information. The printed books were the only valid source of information received. So, cross-checking the facts was presumed as one of the toughest jobs. Normally, words used by senior executives were considered as testimony in itself. Once, while addressing a meeting, some new information was sought. On not getting the correct answer, he got infuriated and shouted –'no one has the correct information'. In the meantime, I entered the room, and before I could gauge the situation inside, he approached me angrily and said that everyone is useless, and no one knows anything. Karl Marx has rightly said, "Man is born free, but everywhere in chains." I without sensing the lull, suddenly and very innocently said that, Sir, it was not Marx, but it was the quote of Rousseau. Breaking the perfect silence, the people standing behind him burst out with laughter. They were the same people who were trying to balance themselves after the accusations leveled at them of being non-knowledgeable. It was the God sent opportunity for them to restore their balance. On hearing this laughter, the manager lost his balance and challenged me to show the source of this information. I was still in shock as I did not know why this challenge was thrown toward me. However, I used my common sense and ruminated on two possible options. Either I should prove myself right by providing him with the right source, thereby disturbing his balance further, or I should maintain calm by not responding to his call and not letting the situation get worsened. So without uttering a single word, I left the room, giving the impression that I had quit. Thereafter, he kept scolding everyone the whole day who came in his way. This continued for three days until I accepted that I could not prove my point. After this, he regained his balance and his behavior turned good with everyone. But, he kept insulting me in every meeting by citing that event in some way or the other. But, I knew I was right and saved the situation for himself and for my colleagues only. So, I had no issue. Further, it was a testing time for me to test my power of tolerance and patience. Rather it was getting strengthened every time he ridiculed me. After completing our tenure, we both got transferred to our requested place.

After almost five years had elapsed, I got his call late at night or in the wee hours, as I remember. Very politely but equally straight, he asked me, "When you could have proved yourself right at that time, why didn't you do it?" I could easily sense that by that time he must have realized that I was right that fine day. That is why he must have been feeling uncomfortable or unbalanced. So, to restore his balance, he wanted to talk to me, admit his mistake, and become balanced. I replied politely, Sir, you were my officer, and if I proved you wrong, you would never have been comfortable in front of me. This could have an adverse effect on your morale and the morale of our organization too. Further, by virtue of being your subordinate, being myself less knowledgeable was not going to affect anyone, if it really did not affect me. I knew that someday you would definitely come out with the truth. Besides, if I could keep myself balanced in every situation, why should I meddle in the costly social investment where there was all loss, no gain? I am still a big fan of you, sir. By thanking each other, we both hung up the call. It was a balancing moment for both of us as whatever the issue with him got a complete ending.

I must be blamed for being reasonably unethical to him by depriving him of the right information at that time. I must say that there is a sea of difference between that time and the right time. Handling the matter that goes public has been one of the most difficult tasks in the universe. If someone feels that he has been insulted publicly, the offender will have to tender an apology publicly or apologize in front of at least as many people, before whom the insult has taken place. Only then will it be considered a solution to the problem. It means if this incident had remained between the two of us only then the situation could have been clarified and sorted out amicably. Further, when any incident takes place, a person is being told publicly that he is wrong; what is actually happening here? In this situation, it is not important who is right and who is wrong. Important to them is what all the people, who thronged around, will think of them. So, there can be no right or wrong answer at that point in time because the problem is not in the frame. The problem is "the four people have heard it or seen it". Now your next bounden duty is to convince those four people that only your own point of view is correct. It means, focusing on convincing those four people instead of focusing on the solution to the main problem is of prime importance. This way, the solution goes berserk, and blaming and counter blaming take their own course, till we get back to the point where we had started. Do we ever get back to the point where we started?

Have you ever seen two people fighting alone in a corner for about an hour? Although you may see two people fighting for a few minutes, at the same time, if a third person arrives, you see their fight gets a new momentum. A similar incident took place when I went to the village school to meet a friend of mine who was working there as a teacher. He took me to the library of his school. Just then, a teacher came rushing towards him and said, "Sir, please come outside, two children are fighting very badly." I also followed them. When I reached the spot I found the information was correct. Two children were fighting severely. Since it was lunchtime, a large crowd of children had gathered to see the duel. Some teachers tried to intervene to get the fighting stopped. The more they tried to intervene, the more aggressive they became, as if they would not rest until they injured each other. One teacher got injured while trying to save another teacher. I was standing quietly with my friend. One of the teachers tried to coerce us to stop them. Suddenly it came out from my mouth "They will stop themselves," and "If you meddle, they will become more aggressive, you simply provide them an uncomfortable condition." I simply asked my friend to get the bell rung as a mark to end lunch time. As soon as the bell rang, the spectator children started going inside their class. During that time the intensity of their fight also gradually decreased. When all the children went inside, both of them stopped as if they had stopped on the orders of a teacher. The teacher who was trying to stop them for the last ten minutes thought that they had stopped on their request. Then both of them stopped fighting and started blaming each other verbally, i. e. instead of a physical fight, they started talking, and finally at the teacher's request, both of them apologized to each other and went into their class. Could this have happened earlier? Yes, but during the time the number of children or people watching them fighting was influencing, making both of them further imbalanced that if they could not do anything, what would that number think about them? This is a state of imbalance and we have taken refuge in it, in perpetuity. This is the situation of today. Believe me, fights and spectators are directly proportional to each other.

To summarize, in our daily life, we use varied forms of energy like anger, humor etc. Actually, these are different combinations of energy, giving birth to thought. Every thought at its subatomic level a pure thought from where it can manifest itself in any form, depending on the efficiency or ability of our choice as its user. As in ray optics or light spectrum, each of its forms has different influencing capabilities as we have seen in the case of M-Tools. In simple words, when we are imbalanced by an external stimulus, we get a literal list of different forms of energy to restore balance, like a dropdown menu on a computer screen. You make the choice, based on your discretion and temperament. Your choice can not be categorized as right or wrong. It will either disturb your balance or achieve a balance. So, always choose an easy and safe option, if you are disturbed. At the same time, analyze the pattern of how others react or respond so that you can keep him also in a balanced state. Now we have discovered that the starting and end point of life is – Peace, the verbatim of balance in all dimensions. Another mystery has to be demystified in the next part, where we discover the way, we achieve the balance by being in the process of communication, the final essence of being human.

Part-III

Communication

Our life is merely a cyclical journey from thought to action. "Simple living, high thinking" has been the universal guiding principle of today's civilized society. As I said in the beginning, our ideas must be high, but the processes through which these ideas are formed have been abstractly explained to us. Different cultures and their literature in the form of philosophy along with our veterans and ancestors have been instrumental in disseminating their own version of the process of formation of thought. Developing high-level ideas is a continuous and conscious process that involves curiosity, critical thinking, creativity, and commitment to lifelong learning. But, this kind of thinking has been a prerogative of only an enlightened group of people that represent only a minuscule section of society.

Therefore, I am not going to address them. They do not need us either. My aim is to make aware the larger section of society, representing the common man who is unable to grasp thoughts directly or to follow the ideas or thoughts of the great personalities of the world. So, following the path of Lord Buddha, "Be a light unto yourself' you can get hold of it through your daily communication style. This is the easiest process to carefully analyze the conversations you do every day. You should have the proper awareness about the type of words and sentences you are using in your day- to -day conversations. You are supposed to enter into conversations with people from diverse backgrounds and viewpoints, listen actively, ask open questions, and participate in discussions. In the process, you must transcend the illusory existence of socially constructed negative and positive people. At its core, people are people, co-humans and you have to interact with them.

Keep in mind that your conversation must be a balanced and smart conversation. Let it be, if it is not effective. There is definitely a difference between effective communication and balanced and smart communication. In effective communication you can influence someone with your eloquence or with your arguments, giving you a feeling that you have convinced them. But, you don't know whether the person on the other side also feels himself balanced in the process. It is possible that he may have a dearth of appropriate words or sentences and be unable to express them under immediate circumstances due to one or the other reason. He may be your subordinate who may not have the courage to express himself before you, despite having better arguments. This way, you force him to vent his frustration somewhere else. If the cycle of balance-imbalance doesn't break somewhere, it will disturb the entire ecosystem of the organizational setting. So for me, it is good that a person in any form of communication balances himself but at the same time, he has to ensure that the person on the other side also achieves a balance so that a cycle of balance-imbalance is broken. So, ensuring balance on both sides is another feature of smart balancing.

I also doubt the role of influencers in ensuring balanced communication. Here we have at least two parties-the influencer and the influenced. Both parties imbalance each other. First, it fuels the overconfidence of the influencer that makes him feel, whatever he says is absolutely correct and can declare any other's viewpoint or argument as ridiculous or baseless. Further, if he finds someone with better logic, he will continuously be trying to influence him further with his sophistry. There are hardly any people who accept other's advice or opinions in this state of overconfidence. Let me cite an incident only to show how balanced communication takes place.

As the head of the institution, I was transferred to a new place. One day an employee came to my office and requested me to listen to his concern. After getting my nod he said, Sir, "Whatever orders you pass, one of our colleagues shows his reluctance to follow your orders that I can't tolerate. So, you should take appropriate action against him."

At the moment, it was not important for me to see whether he was telling the truth or a sheer lie. The pertinent issue was how to respond him. What mattered the most was not to disturb his balance either. Normal behavior demanded I should have gotten angry for showing my eagerness to ask the name of that employee. If I did not respond to him this way, he might have taken me as a feeble officer, which was against the spirit of authority and leadership. It may also be possible that he may have had some difference with that employee, and to balance the imbalance arising out of that difference, he may be using me as a safe tool. I replied, "Sir, the information you have given will be taken care of. Thanks for apprising me of your concern. At the same time, you provided me with the much-needed feedback. Your information has given me a sigh of relief." I further said, "In fact, when I issue an order, I also expect that there should be few who must doubt my order. An organization prospers when these persons come forward and give you feedback, so the remedial steps can be taken in time. Now what matters the most for me is if a person starts following your order unopposed, unquestioned, and rather meekly for fairly a long time without giving any input or feedback, an unhealthy kind of overconfidence have the genesis in you that may go up to the level of narcissism. In the future, you would appreciate that no one should oppose your order in any case, and if someone dares, you will put all your energies into setting them right the way, you want. In that case, your own egoistic interest will rise above the interest of the organization, which will see the growth of the organization stymied." If I look at my entire conversation, the first part of the statement in which I thanked him was to balance him, so that he could not feel that he was giving such an important information and I did not even take cognizance of it. Maybe he was telling the truth or he had a genuine intention. The second part of the statement made him see things a different way around too and it happened exactly. Thereafter, as long as I was there, he worked for the institute with full dedication as a more balanced and enlightened employee.

As far as the person being influenced is concerned, he constantly moves forward to achieve the position of influencer. He will keep longing for chances to retort you back, how you were wrong or at fault. This kind of rivalry has always been common in society. Hence, I believe that our communication should be so organized, immaculate, and balanced that no contrary question arises in the mind of the other person. This way, it opens the door for another new conversation. To achieve this objective, I do emphasize that instead of thinking on the thought first, you should pay attention to your daily conversations, which give rise to your next incoming thoughts. This strengthens your acumen to regulate the already built thought along with the incoming new thought. This will facilitate meaningful and balanced communication.

Communication is the process of sharing information, ideas, experiences, etc. between individuals or groups. Communication can take many forms, such as language, writing, auditory, spoken, visual, and tactile, each of which has its own significance. The main purpose of communication is to share information accurately and clearly so that cooperation and understanding can increase among individuals or groups.

Communication is like a clock, if it does not work properly, you are not able to measure the speed of time and see yourself lagging behind the rest of the world. If we are slow, nothing will be accomplished on time. If we are fast, it will be difficult to maintain harmony with the time. This does not mean that we should not think ahead of time. It means, we should keep our energy replenished and keep pace with the times. Muhammad bin Tughlaq was a great ruler. He has the kudos of undertaking many administrative experiments which were far ahead of his time. It transcended the mental standard of his subjects and all his exemplary experiments failed, if we don't dive deep into different confronting interpretations of contemporary historians.

Our quality of life is based on the nature of choice, we prefer. Every moment we resort to picking and choosing from the available options to stay alive. Even breathing or not is a matter of choice. We are here today because we have not chosen to have stayed there. So, our being in a certain situation is of utmost importance because it's we who have chosen to stay in that situation, sacrificing many other possible situations. So, if you are angry with the person sitting next to you for no reason whatsoever, be careful because it shows that you cannot make the right choice for yourself. When you talk to someone, you think that you are talking to a particular person, but in fact, you are interacting with a situation, and the person involved in communication is serving merely as the carrier of that situation. If we go a little deeper, it is tantamount to answering the questions asked by the situation in a time and space. So, there is no place for judgment or prejudice in a conversation. This does not mean that every situation is completely a new situation. Every color has its dominant color merely by virtue of what is being reflected otherwise, it has all other colors in its core, and our eyes are not designed to see the rest of the recessives. We need not view, but rather visualize the white, the combination of all possible colors. Similarly, we have to prepare ourselves to pierce or see every person, this way, only to reach their core. This will give you the required insight, courage, and confidence to negotiate with varied shades of people in toto. All these are to be expressed through your communication skills in such a way that the target audience can also maintain its balance.

Following are the 6Ps under the three stages of communications, which are understandably essential to achieve this kind of literal balance. Being human, knowingly or unknowingly, we are, by default, a part of the Type B stage of communication. Majority of people live their entire life at this stage only. The majority, out of the rest of the people develop the acumen to enjoy their life by reaching up to the Type V stage. Here, he is able to balance their life considerably. Type H stage is the ultimate stage that only a few can reach. Here, the style of communication matches all the universal values, we cherish in philosophy, but we live in theosophy, where mystical insight is realized in self through the other self and world.

1. Type B Stage

'Type B' stage of communication refers to that stage of communication where a self-centered person enters into any communication with a self-directed purpose. Here his aim is to develop interpersonal relationships for the fulfilment of his/her self-directed goals. This kind of communication is very basic and fundamental to a man who is selfish by nature. That is why I name this style- Type B or Bacterial style of communication, where we lack the elements of universal consciousness and inclination towards objective perception, especially at the initial stage of cognitive development of humans. At this stage, we discuss its three key elements: Person, Purpose, and Perception, but without compromising the soul and spirit of the book, which is 'how to keep ourselves smartly balanced' even at this fundamental stage of communication.

(1) Person

This is the most significant element of communication. Here, a person communicates at three levels-

Communication of a person with himself.

Communication of a person with another person.

Communication of a person with more than one person or with a group.

A person's communication with himself

The orientation or positioning of communication at these three levels is completely different from each other. For example, when a person communicates with himself or it takes place within, he transforms the cosmic energy into a thought meant for him only. We have to admit that his own personality, his socio-economic status, his experiences earned till now and his samskaar or genetic inheritance must have a strong influence in shaping his way of manufacturing the genre of thought and ideas. Let's forget these influences for a while. Additionally, there are myriad types of thoughts, let loose by innumerable sources, reliable or unreliable, received by us, or we mechanically take cognizance and pull thoughts from anywhere, and may be from everywhere, which may be neither yours nor meant for yours. It's simply like a market where varied products are kept, and it's you who have to decide which product you have to choose as per your needs. It's not that you come home with all the products, you see, or simply because handed over to you forcibly by the seller. Similarly, all those thoughts coming from any direction or from whichever address, unchecked and unverified, keep you under stress and anxiety till you process them according to your needs. Here one has to train oneself how to reprocess or reorganize the different nuances of thoughts that are coming in your mind and keep them balanced. You practice a conversational pranayaaam (breathing technique in Ayurveda that involves controlling your breath to connect your body and mind). Let these be entered into your mind, and hold them for a certain period of time to get these reprocessed, balanced and settled into a novel usability. Till the time you live a life of a monarch, because you have complete control over all these thoughts. Once these come out, you turn out it's serf. For rest of your life, it keeps you busy defending, what you say, in terms of present-day terminology it lands you in a position to delete your tweet once it is tweeted. Nevertheless, if you still want to rule over your thoughts, you will have to make sure that your all twitted words make the other person feel balanced and respected too. I am not docile enough to propose the idea of "I win, you win" in any form of conversation. Rather, in that conversation, it's a matter of "to the extent you are in me and I am in you" and for this, it is necessary that along with ensuring the internal balance of your thoughts, you also ensure that the other person is also able to feel the same kind of satisfaction or the same kind of balance from inside.

Once a child asked me, "Sir, how can I become an effective speaker?"

I replied, "It is only, when if you say something to other person and he is not in a position to put up a counter-question."

For a fifteen-year-old child, this was too unambiguous to understand easily.

He said, "Sir, I am confused, you tell me."

I said, "You start the conversation."

He said, "Sir, I want whosoever I talk to he would send a friend request to me instantly."

I asked, "Why? What are the qualities you possess that force others to make friends with you?"

In this way, a counter-question comes up.

He replied back to me, "In this way, how can anyone talk to, if any counter-question does not arise."

I said, "Ok you say, "Namaste" or "Good morning" to someone. Can anyone afford to put counter question, why?"

"At the most, you get in response 'Namaskar' or something similar."

I further added, "You say someone, you are a very intelligent boy in our class. Will they protest or do a counter question, how dare you say as such? Mind your own business."

Here, the question is definitely not, why should I say this? What I mean is when the conversation has the element of respect for a person along with his participation, it will be difficult for anyone to come up with counter-questions. It will only be responded to with equal respect.

A person's communication with another person

When one person enters into communications with you, you have to keep in mind that the person is also in a situation, as I have told you earlier. Person reacts and responds differently in different situations. So, whenever a person talks to you, they talk to you in a given time and space. In each case, his mental state will be different and so will be yours. At 10:30 am, you may be in a good mood, but the other person who has come to talk to you may not be in a good mood. So, you are a situation A, and the other is in situation B. To have balanced and smart communication, at least one has to make sacrifices and come down to the level of the other. So, it is advised that in every situation one should be a good listener. It means, if you want a balanced conversation, first you listen to and get used to the state of mind of others. Now, take a short pause. Organize and reprocess your thoughts accordingly in your mind. Now you say, what you want to say in such a way that makes him feel, that you have listened to him, understood the content, and respond from his position. It's not like you have accepted his viewpoint but it's like you have accepted him as a co-human. You ensure the docking of a wayward ship with a dockyard in the hope of being refurbished. You ensure a connection. It is really great when you connect with him. If you do not want to listen to someone, you definitely listen to him and can express your disagreement politely. Even it is perfectly ethical to maintain animosity without being harsh and disrespectful to your potential enemy and competitors. It's really divine, if you know the art of making foes with love and care. It at least keeps you connected, and nobody knows a one-time enemy may be yours in no time. So, for me, connection is divine. You always see that saying 'no' without establishing a connection will be equivalent to throwing a challenge to someone, and this way you become eligible to get the same treatment from the other side. So, if you want to connect, you follow his pathway. You must have noticed that the process of relationship building is long drawn, spearheaded by the theory of balance.

In my office, I have realized that most of the complaints come to me only because my subordinates did not give complainants time, did not talk to them properly, did not give them the right information, or did not listen to them. Here, whether you do their work or not, is perhaps not as important as the quality or balanced conversation that goes along with it. It's fine, I will not go your way, but it's fine, I am talking to you. For this, I have devised a formula of "2 minutes: 20 minutes". If I know I am not going to do him a favor as it is against the extant rules, I should talk to him for 20 minutes so that he can be convinced, why can I not do this to him? The one whose work I can do, I hardly give him 2 minutes because thereafter, all his words will be in praise of mine. This will render you see more pending work. Further, it will strengthen your belief in expecting that in the future, that person will come back and say thanks to you. But, this hardly happens. Accept it gracefully, you are going to be one of the happiest people in the future. Out of my own experience, whenever I find out that I cannot do favor to someone, I covey the things to him with due respect and open-mindedness. It never happens that the person gives me a frowning look. If he is not happy with me, perhaps he will not have any malice or grudge against me either. And there will be no further reaction, giving a permanent halt to action-reaction dynamics. You achieve a balance, and one episodic cycle is complete.

In most of the cases, I have seen that if a person comes to your office and you are unable to satisfy him because you want to finish the task quickly and do not spare time for him. This disturbs his balance. In the meantime, you don't know that the person sent off dissatisfied from your office is involved in sharing his grievances with like-minded people and his relatives to create further pressure on you to get his work done. There is every possibility that being motivated by those, he will again come to your office, bringing those people along. Your time will be wasted manifold, at least more than before because this time you have to convince the group as a whole. Now, after making the original complainant convinced, it is your responsibility to convince the rest of his associates as well, otherwise, in a short span of time that group pressure can force him back to the original state again, and you see him unbalanced once again. This is also a cyclic process, if a person is unbalanced, he will move towards achieving a balance. If you convince such a person in 20 minutes, it's a great achievement for you, as you have saved much more of your time from being wasted at a later stage of the episode. So, sit comfortably and listen to people, follow the same pathway, reorganize your thoughts, put things in a balanced way and you will see, in the future, they will come only to help you out.

One day, which was probably a very busy day in my office, I was, surrounded by many employees, doing their work one by one. Meanwhile, someone's phone rang. He was probably wishing his wife, who was at her home, 200 kilometers away, on their wedding anniversary.

Upon hearing, I went aloud, "How dare you say this in my presence, in my chamber?"

I didn't know whether it made him scared or not but the immediate and intimidating reaction of rest of the employees, in my favor really made him very scared and he quickly realized that he had committed a blunder.

They all, staring at him started advising, "It was your personal matter and you cannot do this in the chamber of head of the institution. You should apologize immediately."

I was equally bamboozled by the kind of reaction of the rest of the employee. Before the situation goes out of control I wanted to make my intention clear to him.

I told to that employee, "Sir, don't embarrass me further, rather I should be ashamed of myself that I am yet to be accepted by you as yours."

"What I mean to say, either you should have wished your wife far outside my office, keeping me unnoticed to this fact, or you should have told me as such by right, as a token of accepting me as co-human. Now don't waste the best of your time. Take leave and go straight to your home and wish her 'happy marriage anniversary' there only and make it a practice every year."

Can you imagine the level of commitment that he showed thereafter for the organization?

A Person's Communication with more than one or with a group

When a person communicates to a group of people or to a very large group, you may term it as a public address, that too has some requirements. Whenever you speak on such a platform, you need to do a lot of homework on the type of group to whom you are going to address and how these groups will respond to your speech in a balanced manner. Generally we find four groups of audience.

First is the group that will not think logically at all. They believe in whatever you say, unopposed. These are passive groups. Your impact span is for a very short period. After the speech is over, they become inactive, and there will be hardly any possibility of change in them. They need to be motivated again and again. There are chances, if they listen to others on the same day they might agree with them too. Such groups are wonderfully vulnerable and can get excited in other ways also. So, take care to keep them balanced instead of getting them overexcited, otherwise it may not lead to the expected results.

The second group is of those people, who already have some knowledge and they usually compare your statements with their previous knowledge and absorb, as much as, they can and will not absorb, as much as, they cannot. They accept only those ideas that match their preconceived ideas. These people will continue to do the same thing, they have been doing even after listening to you.

The third group consists of those who have not come to listen to you. They take your every word as a challenge and oppose you. Whenever you say something good, they try to disturb you by asking irrelevant questions in between, and want to see you go awry. They know how to rope you in, with their jargon and unverified and unreliable facts and figures. The more you get entrapped, the more you are a matter of pleasure for them. So you are not supposed to be carried away. It is very important to use your words in a balanced way. The most significant characteristic of this group is that, even if they are impressed by you, they will continue to oppose you until they themselves realize their mistake.

The fourth group is the group that accepts you with an open mindedness, invest their time and energy to analyze you, and asks questions, if they have any doubt. They are inquisitive and if convinced they do incorporate your ideas or thought into their lives.

So, whenever you address the public, you must believe in the theory of balance. Your script should be all-inclusive. There should be at least something for all these four groups in order to make them balanced. The words to be used must enthuse respect for all the classes of the audience. They will listen to you better with equal respect.

As I delineated earlier, how to guard whether your conversation or address is balanced. Trail the path of your audience and reach the root of their thinking. Then, adjust your content accordingly. Strategically, it is like catching them from behind when they are in their comfort zone and become ready to accept you and your thought. They will not deliver, till they accept you in a balanced way.

I recall an incident when I was addressing a batch of trainee educators. One of them, representing the group wanted me to endorse what he thought was right, but I could not support his stand because it was inherently unscrupulous. He was representing group three of the audience as explained above.

He asked, "Sir, what could be the measures to be taken to bring those children on the right path, who are not ready to listen to us?"

I said, "Explain to them."

They said, "Even then, if they do not understand"?

I said, "Explain to them politely."

They fought back, "Sir, what should we do if they still do not understand?"

I said "Explain to them again." Now, if you reach to the sub atomic level of this kind of thinking, you can easily catch hold of it. Actually he wanted me to say that scolding and beating children is essential to bring them on the right track.

I replied again, "If they still ignore your piece of advice or instructions and not coming on the right track, you have to see that you lack essential inputs. Win their trust. Ask their real problems, understand them, talk to their parents and then act accordingly."

He said, "Sir, if they still do not understand?"

I said, "There might be a flaw in your content and the way you are explaining things to them."

"Rethink and change your method of counseling. You also need introspection."

Till now, he himself became tired of his own style of talking and ultimately came to his main point and said,

"Sir, don't you think scolding and physical punishment can bring the desired change in them?"

This way I brought him here so that I could get an entry point into his way of thinking. This access helped me to land on my destination, but the passage I chose, was his only. By now, I was convinced that no matter what my view was on the issue, he would not agree with me, and even if he agreed, he would not implement it in real life. Now it was pertinent for me to follow his pathway and I did. This was the only way to make him come around to the gravity of the issue that he himself raised.

Now, as soon as I yielded to his viewpoint by giving the statement "If you feel that all your ways have failed to bring him on the right path then you can. In this way, you can also save your valuable time and energy."

Now he got what he wanted and felt himself balanced. He took his seat calmly as there was no further question for him to put. This way, by proving his intellectual prowess he could establish a collective balance amongst the whole group of participants too. I could hear the sound of group satisfaction in the form of clapping they did thereafter. But I had not finished yet. I only reached his sojourn and I was supposed to get back to my home too.

I further said, "After resorting to your own method of reformation the biggest responsibility of yours begins from here."

They asked, "What type of responsibility, sir?"

I asserted, "Now, you must start tracking and monitoring their entire life pathways, and it must be you only to ensure that during the entire course, the children do not come on to the right path. There must not be any improvement in them."

They all thought that it might have been a "slip of the tongue."

He replied back, "Sir, if they don't improve, what is the rationale behind resorting to that kind of punishment."

"Yes, I mean it." I continued.....

"This is because after getting this kind of punishment, if improvement in the children take place, they will definitely learn one thing, giving physical punishment is the only way to bring desired results. So, for the rest of their life, wherever they will go, in whatever situation or position they will be, they have learned, if any improvement is to be brought about, this is the only path to be followed. Now you think, being an educator, what kind of product are you sending to society. But, if they are brought on the right path after a lot of hard work, investing your time in explaining them continuously with love and care, what kind of message of love will they take to society? So, now it is up to you, what kind of pathway you are creating for the future generation of our society." The applause that followed must have been ten times more this time than before. So decode the purpose of the group and convey to them whatever is right and ought to be taught with your full commitment, determination, patience, and balanced way. Here, the matter of discussion should not be what the previous generation used to think. If you are addressing the present generation, we have to be amenable to the thought pattern of the present generation which is to the fore with all its merits and demerits. No matter how much time and energy it takes.

(2) Purpose

Every person involved in communication must have a purpose. But the definite and ultimate purpose is to keep oneself in balance. In general, you see that whenever you have a meeting, you have its agenda in place. A person definitely divulge the purpose of his communication either at the beginning or in the middle, or at the end of the conversation at his convenience. In daily chores of life, if someone comes to us, we generally and mandatorily ask, "Tell me, why have you come?" Whenever a subordinate or employee comes to see his officer, he has to assume that he must have some purpose. It is also seen when someone meets you, he may say, "I only just came to meet you." This also carries a definite purpose. He may be feeling bored or he needs to be refreshed after long working hours. Spending some time with you may give him some rest, so that he is back to work afresh. Sometimes the purpose of the ongoing conversation is revealed in the third or fourth round of the conversation. Different types of people cleverly pull out their purpose from their sleeves at the point most convenient to them. They also choose the manner in which they should come up with a purpose. Some by laughing, some by making others laugh, some by praising you, and some by appealing, and so on. A central idea in any communication is that the sooner one comprehends the purpose, the better one will be able to regulate the entire course of communication.

Some people habitually want to keep themselves always at the center of any communication as if no one else matters. They think, when they are free, others will also be free. When they are awake, others also must be awake. Today, you can check your friends' messages on WhatsApp anytime. If he is awake at 3 am in the morning, he can forward you a good morning message with a shaking cup of tea without realizing that you might be sleeping, and the message tone can disturb your precious sleep. He can call you anytime, without asking whether you are available to talk at the moment.

I remember an incident during my hostel days. It was a time when I was doing my graduation. I was allotted my room right next to the Washroom. Initially, it was a blessing in disguise as I used to rise late. But soon the myth was broken. My room turned into a restroom for all my co-hostellers who, while going to or passing through the washroom, invariably prefer to spend some time in my room, not necessarily with me. They can see many more things in the room other than me. Like biscuits, audio cassettes, latest magazines, my new pair of shocks, can be used by them for their use, initially on loan, not to be returned in the future. If I am having breakfast they can take it away with them to be had after taking a bath. Honestly speaking, it did real damage to my study pattern. To make your understanding very clear, I narrate here about a sample Sunday evening. I sit to study at 6 pm. One of my friends, after visiting the washroom came and wasted an hour of my time and went away. At 7:00 pm, another one came and sat down for another hour. Perhaps he had come from the market, he also told the story of his shopping for an hour. Thereafter, he tendered his genuine apology that his intention was not to disturb me. Actually, he had to go to the washroom, and he saw my door open. So he came to say hi-hello. Similarly, everyone comes at their own convenience and weathered hours of my precious time. One reported in my room at 10 pm. On being asked, I came to know that he had been studying since 6 pm, he was feeling tired and thought of having a chat with me to lighten his mind. After that, one more came at 12 am. His issue was really revolutionary. He shared his genuine reason, why he came to my room at this odd hour. He had slept from 6 pm to 12 am and would now sit to study for the next three to four hours. In that case, he would rise late in the morning. So to avoid his late arrival in the class the next morning, he had come to the washroom to shave his beard.

I told him, being unnecessarily harsh on him, "Then, do and go".

He replied innocently, "Water is not coming into the washroom."

So, till water comes he decides to chat with me. In all these cases nobody afford to show interest in knowing my needs. If I oppose, it would have attracted collective opposition and it was difficult to face a social boycott in hostel. So, from now onwards I cooperated with them, started to keep some magazines and light eatables in my room, so that at least I could get some time to study.

It is said that likeminded people live together. Is it still so? Shouldn't we think that people only with similar purpose can live together and that too, till the time they feel that their purpose can be achieved only with each other's cooperation?

(3) Perception

Perception is the act of organizing, identifying, and interpreting sensory information so that the information presented can be understood correctly. All perception involves signals passing through the nervous system, which in turn results from physical or chemical stimulation of the sensory system. Perception plays a very important role in keeping the communication process balanced. If you know the purpose of communication well and rightly perceive the person involved in communication and at the same time you are being perceived rightly by your co-communicator, balanced communication is bound to take place. Perception helps us to build a certain type of impression on the basis of which the communication process is continued. Impression formation is the result of two step authentication process. Through senses or physical mode and through the mental image or metaphysical mode.

Through the senses

Through our senses, the external stimulus prepares us to experience the things that exist outside in the physical world. We have eyes to see the world around us, ears to hear, noses to smell invisible, tongues to taste, and skin to feel the touch. Apart from its functional roles, the very structure and location of the sense organs is the testimony in themselves, how nature has silently explained how these are to be used in a balanced way. Our two eyes symbolize a balanced vision. Your eyelids provide you the freedom to decide what you want to see and what you do not want to see. Two ears convey the message of nature that we should listen to both sides. This can be called balanced listening. Now, what is the difference between eyes and ears? You do not have the freedom to see everything, but there is no constraint on listening. Ears have no gates at all. You are free to listen to sound or noise, coming from any direction. That is why we have to develop the art of listening. There is nothing like the art of seeing. Now, if you look at your nose, here also you will find two gates to balance the breath. You are able to use it when the thing comes closer to you.

As far as the tongue is concerned, it is one of the finest structural marvels of our sensory system. It is strategically located under the security cover of two natural barriers. One is like a soft gate and another is like portcullis. Our lips are that soft gate that is usually closed. This insinuates that before you speak, you first have to make some effort to open the Lips' gate or lip gate. Thereafter, you see an iron gate, in the form of teeth under which the tongue is locked. This is more like a portcullis. These are all to remind you, that the source of your words is like a bank locker which is safely placed inside a soft and an iron door that you can use only when it is absolutely necessary. Further, look at the softness, flexibility, and suppleness of the tongue, which indicates that even if the situation worsens, it can be corrected through balanced communication by bringing the required change in communication flow.

The two nostrils of the nose play an important role in balancing our entire mind-body system through Pranayama. Now, if you look at your skin, it makes you feel things much closer to you and helps those who cannot identify the things through any other mediums, i.e. eyes and ears.

So, the collective design of the sense organ serves as a motherboard of our communication system. Its architecture, provides two clear messages of nature. First, you have to listen to everyone, as much as you can, but when you speak, think a thousand times before. The reason is that every word that emanates from your mouth is the input, the raw material for others, on the basis of which a person can form thousands type of ideas for himself in the process of ongoing communication. It is of paramount importance, "Will it be able to balance them all, who participate in the communication process?" Or it will make them unbalanced, leaving them to react ad infinitum to regain balance. It is our responsibility to oversee and regulate the whole process of communication in a balanced way.

Through mental imagery

So, it is necessary that your perception about things or people is correct. You should use all the five senses correctly. It should also be ensured that you are in a position to satisfy all the five senses of the other parties involved in the conversation. If I talk about interpersonal relationships, it means to connect. Connecting means acceptance. If there is acceptance, then to what extent? The more accepting you are, the more you are able to connect with co-communicators. But, it must take place both ways. To make things easier, see the example. If someone likes your appearance, it is to be considered that your acceptability is 20%. If they enjoy listening to you, your acceptability is enhanced by 20% more. Similarly, if you are decent-looking with good speaking and listening skills, your acceptability is enhanced to 20% + 20% = 40%. Again, if the location where you are talking is clean, hygienic, and fragrant, then add 20% more. When you hold a meeting for a discussion or invite someone to your home and you serve them good food, your acceptance probability will further increase by 20%. If you meet warmly with a warm handshake, then add 20% to this as well.

So, it means total acceptance is acceptance through all five senses. In this case you are able to converse in a better and balanced manner. Here, I would like to make it clear that this percentage is only for understanding the example. Its ratio is a variable that depends on the mental maturity of the person. So, to satisfy the eyes, you should look decent, to satisfy the ears, use good words, to satisfy the nose, you should talk in a clean and hygienic ambiance, and for rest of the two senses, arrange sumptuous food, and welcome with full warmth by warm shaking hands or the way the cultural customs of the place demands. You will see, your conversation will get a better orientation. You can see, how important meetings are conducted. You can continue in this order, on the availability of resources under your command, till your purpose is achieved. So, in any conversation, you should know the demands note of the five senses. According to the demand note of the eyes, you should appear good. Keep yourself organized as you are, dress and body posture should be appropriate to the time and space. Your decent looks are your first impression. Here, looks have nothing to do with how one perceives. It is about universal goodness, how you present yourself on the occasion. Further, use decent words in a balanced way in the conversation that must be pleasant to the ears. This does not mean that you should say only what they like to hear but also what they ought to hear. At the same time, say not only what they ought to hear but also what they like to hear. Along with the choice of good and balanced words, if the communication style, tone, pause, and non-verbal communication are in the right configuration, this can be called your second impression. For the third, fourth, and fifth impressions, you can see the example mentioned above. For the sixth and last impression, you will have to depend on the mental image of the listener who reacts by rearranging, modifying, and processing the data, received from the five senses according to the time and situation.

2. Type V Stage

The name of this stage of communication is coined due to the features the Viruses possess. Viruses demonstrate reprogramming capabilities by manipulating things for their own replication and perseverance. These features allow viruses to establish and maintain their influence over time. This feature we expect to be adopted by all the parties who enter into conversations through reprogramming with an aim to serve the universal principle of keeping things smartly balanced.

(4) Program

Here I mean 'Program' as 'mental program.' "Mental programming" in communication refers to the process of shaping or influencing a person's thoughts, beliefs, and attitudes through various forms of communication. It involves using language, symbols, and messages to influence the way people understand information, events, or ideas.

Effective mental programming involves crafting messages that match the feelings, values, and cognitive processes of the audience. This can influence decision-making, shape opinions, and contribute to the formation of attitudes.

When a person forms an assumption, keeping his purpose in mind, his assumptions keep changing during conversations with other people. It is very easy to form an assumption about a person whom you have never met or talked to because in that case, there are absence of inputs or having unreliable and distorted inputs. You make notions in your mind according to your convenience and keep carrying them throughout your life. For example, if someone sees you and does not greet you, you may feel that he is arrogant.

Once a child of grade one complained to me by pointing to his classmate "Sir, he abuses me."

I asked his classmate, and he denied it.

Again, the child added, "No sir, he is lying, he abuses me."

Once again, I asked his classmate, "Why do you do this to him?"

The classmate reasserts, "No sir, I am saying the truth, I don't lie. I never used a slang against him."

Both appeared to be so true. So, I called some of their other classmates.

I asked them all, "Who is saying the truth"?

They all said, "We have never seen these two talking anymore."

Finally, I asked the complainant child, "You let me see by imitating him how he abuses you."

He finally, with all his innocence, comes to a great answer "Sir, he slangs me in his mind."

This is not only a case of children, this is the case with all of us. This happens when there is a communication gap among the parties involved. Sometimes this gap becomes so big that we end up creating a story of two generations. If we look at the last two world wars, one of the main reasons was no dialogue between the two blocks. Both felt that whatever one was doing was against the other block. This is why there should be no gap in dialogue if you are intended to resolve issues. It is better to maintain communication till trust is restored. So, keep your mind flexible enough and keep reviewing the situation. Keep looking for as many inputs as possible and never form a closing opinion. There is no need to form a final opinion too, to live. If someone talks to you a lot someday, you form the notion that he is very talkative. As you spend more time with him, you guard your relationship for a considerable period of time and enjoy a much longer relationship. During this time, not only does it become difficult for you to form a definite opinion, but you also need to change the opinion that you had formed earlier about him. So, as you are in a longer relationship or in a longer conversation, you will have to adjust your opinion time and again, believing in the notion, as told earlier, that you see a person but interact with a situation. So, perception is bound to be dynamic. As our perception changes, the orientation of our conversations will also change, leading to changes in responses too. It means, we should not be in a hurry to form any opinion. We need to study all the inputs that we receive from various sources. This is what we call programming or reprogramming.

(5) Perseverance

Perseverance in communication refers to the ability to persist, endure, and maintain efforts in communicating a message, especially when faced with challenges or obstacles. This often involves making sure the message is clear and easily understood.

Once I had a fever. It was 11:00 pm.

My wife sensed my pulse like a doctor and said, "It was 104 degrees Fahrenheit."

Since I was feeling fine, I replied, "It cannot be more than 101 or 102."

My wife took it as a challenge. She now put the thermometer under my tongue to take a fresh reading. It was a little dark and she was also tense, so, wrongly read it 105. 5 degrees Fahrenheit.

I, giving her a frowny look, said, "This is not possible."

I can easily sense the tension she had on her face. She, with her trembling hand, picked up the thermometer to take the measure once again, but it fell down and broke. She became even more tense now. What would she do, if it needed late night? She decided to get a new thermometer from her parents, who lived about 5-6 km away from my residence. In a nervous and trembling voice, she called them and informed them that I had a fever of 105 degrees and the thermometer was broken, come immediately. When her parents heard, they became even more worried. They rushed to my home in no time, but without getting a new thermometer.

She surprisingly asked, "Where is the thermometer?"

They gave their perplexed look said, "You should have told me."

In fact, she mixed two different sentences into one. She meant that I had a fever of 105 degrees and the thermometer at home was broken, so they should come with a new thermometer. I knew this or she knew it. But for them, it was like the thermometer broke due to soaring body temperature. The first part of the sentence made them so tense, that they could not even recall the common sense science. In this way, if you are not able to talk or communicate clearly, the person on the other end of the conversation corrects the information in his own way, irrespective of being involved in the philosophy of right or wrong. Most of the rumors and misunderstandings take root from this kind of half-cooked communication.

In the process of conversation, active listening and the willingness to listen actively involves- accepting the other person's perspective and adapting communication strategies, as needed. This demonstrates a commitment to understanding and responding appropriately in the appropriate time and space. It is critical to maintain flexibility in communications, adapting communication styles to suit different types of audiences in dynamic situations or addressing unexpected challenges. Building understanding and acceptance when facing resistance, requires finding alternative ways to deliver the message or address concerns.

For example, once a person came to my office. He was very angry. He was probably not happy with the behavior of one of my subordinates. He was venting all his anger on me. I was listening to him quietly. Perhaps my silence and non-reacting approach challenged him even more. The truth was that during his unstoppable utterances, I was waiting for the right time to enter when he would not feel challenged when I responded. So, I intentionally delayed my response time. I still maintained my silence. My constant silence disturbed his balance.

He got angry and challenged, "Sir, let me tell you, I have connections with many high ups, I can do anything."

I swiftly sneaked politely, "Sir, don't lie, you cannot do everything," and without wasting a second, I added, "If you can do anything and everything, you can forgive my employee too. Do you think you can do this?" I continued.

"Either you forgive him or take your statement back." In response he smiled lightly on my witty but respectfully convincing circumlocutory remarks that completed a cycle of conversation with an amicable solution.

Balanced communication requires patience and bringing reasonable change in communication stance, especially in complex or sensitive situations. Be it personal relationship, professional settings, or public speaking, persistence is a valuable quality that contributes to building understanding, trust, and successful communication outcomes. It includes a continued commitment to the communication process even when faced with difficulties or resistance.

3. Type H Stage:

This is the final stage of communication where we enter into any communication with an aim to merge the individual identity with universal identity in the interest of establishing a collective balance that is in consonance with the ultimate mandate of this Universe. That is why I call it a Type H stage or Human stage. All the processes adopted at the first two stages got crystalized here in perpetuity. Reaching this stage will not only make you a smart communicator, and wonderful motivator but also a life-maker of self and other selves.

(6) Projection

Switchboard Model of Communication

Till now we have studied how a person enters into communication with his surroundings. How to get hold of purpose, invariably implicit in any form of communication, along with comprehending the structural and locational characteristics of the sense organs and their demands. How to make necessary adjustments in our perceptions and get it reprogrammed as per the requirement. At the same time, we could know the obstacles we face during the process of communication and follow the rule of persistence and patience. Now the question is how we can carry our viewpoint to the other side of our co-communicators so that not only the self, but they too, become balanced. Our cardinal objective has always been to make balanced, meaningful, and smart communication possible. As it is already asserted apart from a person, a person is also a situation. So, whenever you talk to a person, first delve deep into their inner self to get apprised of the firsthand information on the situation in which one exists. Here lies the importance of Switchboard model.

We all human beings are the model of a virtual switchboard. How does it happen, a person is definitely better able to convince others and can also be convinced when explained to them by others. At the same time, the other person can neither convince anyone nor be convinced when explained to them by others. Let us understand it this way. Every conversation entails an action–reaction continuum or equation that follows a certain pattern. Whenever a person speaks, the other person reacts or responds in three ways. Either he cooperates, or he challenges, or he remains neutral or indifferent. The conversation is like a switchboard. Imagine you have an electric switchboard, fixed in a new room with 10-12 switches, fixed thereon. Each switch is exclusively assigned to run fans, bulbs, and night bulbs. But, if you are using it for the first time and you do not know how the switches are connected with each other, there is always a greater probability of switching on the wrong one. If you want to switch on a fan, you get to see a bulb gets on. You want to switch on a bulb, you see a fan is on, and if it is winter season, there are more chances of the fan being switched on. Most of the time, you start from the first switch and try after the second, third, and fourth, you get success by reaching upto the last switch, provided the bulb and the connections are correct.

Similarly, whenever a conversation fails onus is on the doer. He constantly chooses the wrong switch, and before he reaches the right one, he falters, leaving the conversation aborted midway. Have patience, try to go deep into the conversation, and keep searching for the right switch. You are sure to find out during the conversation if you are fully alert, neutral, and patiently involved in the conversation. First of all, when you engage a person in a conversation, his first question or the way he enters into the conversation will give you decisive hints, on what direction he wants to take the conversation. So the first principle is that you have to start in the direction he wants.

So, the first principle is, you have to start in the direction the other wants. If you oppose or resist him in the beginning, it will be difficult for you to establish the much-required connection till the end of the conversation. For the success of the conversation, it is necessary to first establish a relationship with your co-communicator. Once your relationship is established, you can take the conversation forward. As your conversation progresses, be observant of all his cues or response, verbal or non-verbal. For example, if you are saying something to him and you see he is listening, but it doesn't affect his body language. His eyelids are down, or he is playing with the object lying on the table, or looking here and there, which means he has nothing to do with what you are saying. This is the wrong switch you are playing with. So, change the switch immediately. This time, also if you receive the same response, go to the third switch. Minute and negligible change in verbal or nonverbal response doesn't give you enough hints. It might be a courtesy response, like 'hmm', or 'ok'. So, change the topic or the method. At any moment, if you observe a sudden change in his physical posture or mental alertness, like suddenly moving from his place or straightening his waist or widely open eyelids or raising his head and looking straight into your eyes, this is the time of realization that you have pressed almost the right switch. Now you can continue the conversation in that direction till you reach its final goal of the conversation.

There is also a possibility, that you may not reach the final conclusion and come to a stalemate. Once again, we are back to our ongoing conversation. If the reaction is in the form of some harshness or rudeness or verbal disagreement, admit that you have pressed the loose switch that can cause a short circuit. First, you experience resistance through non-verbal signals. Then come words expressing his disagreement. Stop the conversation immediately. Even then, you continue, he might get angry. If it still continues, he will deny or disprove your point. Now the time has come, you stop the conversation immediately and ask for time or change the topic and leave it for today.

If you continue even now, earlier he was against your utterances, now he would oppose and challenge your entire personality. After this, your conversation can go awry in any direction. It will also affect your future relationship. So, keep an eye on the indicators, which are his verbal and non-verbal cues. The switches are his issues of concern or difference and the regulator, by which the speed of the fan is regulated, you can regulate your action-reaction dynamics by looking at the verbal and non-verbal signals of the conversation. This way, following this switchboard model of conversation, you can establish a balance in communication. This will not only improve your relations with all but also make it easier for you to achieve everything in life by giving the right balance of self with self, and self with others, and this way you attain the eligibility to be in line with the ultimate goal of the supreme energy –The Universe.

At last I am citing an incident reminding me of a wonderful communicator who had all the elements of balanced thought and balanced communication. I was once traveling on a train. Two unknown passengers have been talking to each other for the past half an hour. Suddenly, they got involved in heated arguments, and a person called the other person 'saala'. In normal circumstances, it literally means "wife's brother," but in some parts of our country, if used out of disrespect or anger by people, who have no family relation with each other, it is considered as slang, highly disrespectful, and humiliating.

First, what must be the mental state of the first person when he called the other person 'saala'. He must have got angry with him. If he had controlled his anger, he would not have used the word 'saala' against him. Now, when the first person called the other 'saala', it became a matter of self-respect for him. How would the rest of the co-passengers think of him if he didn't do something against him? He also has to tell the crowd that he is no less than the first person. This way his balance was disturbed. Without choosing a word in response, he used his physical strength to nudge him ferociously and said, 'How dare you to call me 'Saala'?

Both parties entered into a serious clash. All the passengers in the bogie felt panicky. Soon, the situation became out of control. We could all expect at any moment it could usher in a violent clash. Meanwhile, an elderly person from amongst co-passengers intervened, who turned out to be instrumental in ending the dispute at its root. Here you witness how a person with expertise in conversation turned the situation upside down in favor of the common good.

The old man started with, "What is the matter?"

Second Passenger said angrily, "Just see his audacity, he called me Saala."

First Passenger pleaded, "But, first he provoked me."

The old man asked- "Is Saala an abuse?" "I do not know. My brother-in-law calls me Saala."

Second passenger: "He was your Jija (brother-in-law in English) hence, he called you 'Saala'. Since he is not my jija he has no right to address me as 'Saala'."

The old man said, "How do you call this woman of your age sitting next to you?"

Second passenger: "I am from a decent family. I call all unknown women as sister or didi (elder sister)."

The old man: "So, unknowingly you might have called this person's wife as sister or didi. In return, he called you "Saala" today. So, it should not be a matter of any dispute. Suppose you have not met his wife till date, if you meet his wife right now, would you call her didi or bhabhi?"

People understood what the old man said. Both the people who were involved in the fighting gave a pretty smile at the old man. The old man was convincingly controlling the rhythm of his conversation. He turned towards the person who had abused him. But this time, with a bit acidic, asked "What harm did that person do to you, that you had put all your sanskar or ancestral value at stake." The person who had abused him felt ashamed. He realized his mistake and apologized to the other person. In return, the other person jokily said, "Today I will have to complain against you to my sister." On this, all burst into a laughter. This event made the rest of the journey for all the passengers traveling in the bogie memorable. How do you rate the entire conversation? Don't you think that a right and smart communicator can give the situation the right direction?

There is yet another dimension of this incident required to be understood. Why does one choose to go slang? It has two premises. One, the person who abuses is weak, has a dearth of appropriate words and cogent logic, sans intellect and wisdom. He is fragile and vulnerable to external stimuli and loses balance easily. He is not enlightened enough to choose the right options as the situation demands. That is why he abused. You must have often seen that when caught lying, not getting their point across, or running away from the situation, people lose their balance and choose anger because they have no other option available. By getting into a state of anger, they gain immense energy and do something unwarranted, for which they have to pay a heavy price later. Whereas a balanced person, like the old man you saw, acted with restraint. He used his energy judiciously and regulated the situation according to his wishes. Therefore, to recombine your energy in adverse circumstances, select that energy combination from the dropdown menu in the larger interest of self and other selves.

Generally, choosing anger in its different forms is the easiest option available to us in case we fail to respond to a situation. How these have been going on since time immemorial? In order to get your balance back, you need to respond. Since you don't have access to M-tools from the dropdown menu, you rely on what you have been trained for years. It is either to control your anger or to burst out. It is a way to let the pent-up feeling come out to get one relaxed. This has been practiced for a long. Rather, we have been taught that 'showing anger or being angry' is the most natural and socially sanctioned response in case we are disturbed.

It is very simple. You merely need to know, what this book stands for. The balance is the ultimate authority. You respond to a situation in response to your balance being disturbed. You are disturbed by a certain combination of energy. So, you get your balance back by recombining the energy, conducive to restoring the required balance. This may be called the reverse osmosis of energy. I suggest you follow a novel Recombinant E-technology. This is a process of energy engineering that uses various mental techniques to isolate and manipulate energy combinations by taking cognizance of the energy spectrum as discussed in part two of this book. The overall aim is to reduce energy toxicity and the associated side effects and to achieve greater stability of human thought and human response, where the way you express yourself to a situation holds the key. Now you crack the competitive examination easily, you excel in academics. You achieve insurmountable heights in the corporate world, you become a leader in whatever field you want. You become everything you want and you live the way you choose, but everything without compromising your health and wealth, mental, physical, and spiritual well-being. You see, how bacteria, viruses, fungi, or algae grow to their full potential only under different and specific ranges of pH, temperature, and moisture. So is the case with vegetation growth. You can't grow everything everywhere as all need a favorable condition to grow naturally while keeping all its desirable properties intact. You reverse the condition and see the results reversed.

We humans are also not an exception to it. We all, too need a favorable condition to grow to our full potential. Smart balancing is a process to create a state of balance. This state varies from person to person depending upon their own time and space. This is the state which we call the most favorable climate for anyone to grow to realize one's full potentials. So, dear friends, "No Emotions, Its all about smart balancing-its all about Life In-Out." Your runway is ready now, wishing you a perfect take off…..

Author's Note: Key Takeaways

I think, therefore I am at ease. I think, therefore I have the disease and I overthink therefore, I am self-displeased.

We all want to be healthy for which we can choose a healthy life style. We change our food patterns, do yogic exercises, or go for a walk daily, resorting to naturopathy. We all know this fact, and we all know that we should and we can lead a healthy life. But the majority of us will never do it voluntarily, however, some start under pressure and will put a final full stop once the motivation level comes down, and still some can continue due to medical reasons.

In short, everybody wants to lead a healthy lifestyle but has no time at all. I hereby propose a novel therapy– "Communication Therapy" for which we don't have to spare extra time nor have to take extra pressure, as being a human, we are very much in communication naturally. We all speak, we all can hear, we all can think. But the only change will be what, why, how, when, and where the communication takes place, leading to balanced communication. This is for those who have no time to adopt the lifestyle as mentioned above.

If I ask a person how did you get High Blood pressure or Diabetes? Most of them will say, we have a lot of work pressure, a lot of tension that I am not performing. To relieve the pressure, we can start taking medicine, falling into some kind of intoxication or addiction which further deteriorates the condition and will take us too far from getting a solution. I am not taking the case of an accident or genetic disease. I am to deal only with those ailments that are directly associated with simply thinking, underthinking (not up to one's potential) or overthinking that don't come out in the form of communication or action, making things imbalanced.

Now, what is your communication pattern? You don't want to talk to, and in place you feel depressed, showing anger or irritation. You simply think about what people think of you, and although they may not be thinking of you, you don't discuss it with them, though you choose to discuss it with others. So, observe your pattern of communication. If under the raze of anger, you hit someone who is socially, politically, and economically more powerful than you, what do you think after one hour? Perhaps it will put you under a lot of tension out of impending fear, at least for the next few days. If you hit someone who is weaker and poorer than you in many aspects, you may feel pity on yourself that you should not have done with that poor fellow. However, you have the option to remain indifferent, but it's very difficult for a normal human being.

In this book, I am not dealing with the case of habitual and hardcore offenders. My address is to at least 70% of the people who own various lifestyle diseases due to bad communication style. So, the purpose of this book is to endorse a concept of "balanced communication" and whenever you do this, you take it as a therapy. Follow the ideas of this book, talk to your enemies, talk to your friends, talk to everybody, if you get an opportunity with equanimity, irrespective of any prejudices, and enjoy your life, see how you feel the resonance of universal energy in you. Only peace- no disturbance. This leads you to achieve everything that you want in life. Now you have no anger, no jealousy, no violence, you don't fight, you talk of the growth of self and of others. Now, know the Absolute reality-Balance and have it achieved through balanced thought, which in turn through balanced and smart communication.

Whenever we fall ill, feel stressed, or not in a good state, we find a way to get out of it. We do yoga, see the doctor, take medicines, or get help from different systems of medicine. Does it ever happen, when we are in a good state, happy or healthy, we try to get out of it? Definitely not. At the most, we may worry that these days should not be of shorter duration. This way, we have a unique kind of Unwellness Cycle. We can divide the cycle into three phases:

1. *Condition before being stressed or falling into illness:*

We take preventive measures to ensure not get into stressed. Most of the people push themselves too much to be healthy throughout their life. This also creates a kind of stress.

2. *Condition during stress or illness:*

You tend to investigate the cause of stress or getting sick. "Which medicine and lifestyle suits you better?" You don't trust your doctor. In place, you search on Google. Most of the time, you pick the most dreaded kind of stress and disease for yourself and keep the other members of your family under stress. You may think, now you can't come out of it. You are lagging behind at your work place and become a storehouse of similar kind of thoughts. Now you choose to remain stuck to it 24x7.

3. Condition after the stress is over, and you get well, you are waiting for the condition when you fall ill or get stressed again:

The moment we recover, we go unbridled and are back to the same lifestyle in which we were before. This way our life continues to be in this cycle, in perpetuity, in such a way that stress or illness or unwellness becomes the ultimate truth. This may be interrupted by a brief period of happiness, but there is every possibility you fall prey to the first and second phases once again to find the vicious cycle of unwellness going on well.

Now, if we are to be always in stress or distress only, how nice it would be if we didn't need to take medicine separately. In place of taking medicine separately or seeing a doctor, reorganize our lives in such a way that every action of ours becomes equivalent to taking medicine. It's like, we are constantly in a healing process, as if being in a healthy state, is itself a state of illness.

It is this kind of healing process that I am talking about in this book. This healing process is our daily conversations that we engage in every day, willingly or unwillingly. We can all experience in our day-to-day life that most of our illnesses or stress are bred out amidst our everyday conversations. You see that if you remain silent, you are free from many stresses. Speaking less than necessary will keep you under stress. Speaking more than necessary will keep you under stress. Saying the right thing at the wrong place will keep you stressed. Talking without keeping in mind the right space and time will keep you stressed. Using the right words or sentences in the wrong way will also keep you stressed. Our stress and tension are the most unguarded gateway through which almost all kinds of diseases get safe passage to one's organic system which has been challenging our physical and mental health. Apart from this, our risk of getting sick and organic deformities can also be due to accidents or genetic causes. If we ignore this, then about 70% of the reasons for getting stressed or getting sick are related only to the fact that we do not take our daily conversations seriously, or are associated with the way we are dealing with information. From today onwards, you should accept that whenever you talk, you are taking medicine or are undergoing treatment. Take this- 'Talking is like taking medicine'. What I mean to say is that when we fall ill and are on medicine, we are much more disciplined. If we show the same kind of discipline in our daily conversations, you will see that you are bound to be healthy, strong, and capable of doing everything that keeps you ahead in your life. You may name it a conversational discipline. It will save you from unwarranted deviation and uncalled for complications arising out of, out-of-place communication or "conversational tension" wherein most of the time we are engaged in. This automatically sets you free from the clutches of the fruitless communication web. This paves the way for you to make yourself a 'focused self and focused co-human'. Here you have full awareness of the work ecosystem in which you live – This is a key to success for all who desire to utilize the best they have.

From today, prepare yourself to be in communication therapy. Realize the power of balance as described in the second part of this book and use the drop-down menu properly as suggested therein. Get hold of the 6Ps suggested in the third part and rely on the switchboard model of communication. This whole process will expand your energy by keeping you with yourself and yourself with other-selves. In other words, it has the capacity to expand your interpersonal relationship to infinity. The more this relationship expands, the more energy you are able to store and use when needed. This process will help you to unearth your infinite potential and award you the courage and confidence to use it in such a way that you can scale the highest peak of life. This is all about "Life in – out", the epitome of universal balance that is to be achieved.

Thank you for being connected. Wishing you to achieve, whatever is achievable with your healthy body and peaceful mind.

www.ingramcontent.com/pod-product-compliance
Lightning Source LLC
La Vergne TN
LVHW041937070526
838199LV00051BA/2820